Sex Games For Couples

Spice up Your Life as a Couple
With Erotic Games; Role Play
Games; Toys and Many Other Dirty
Games to Change Your Normal
Routine and Increase Intimacy in
Your Relationship

Tatiana Stafford

Table of Contents

INTRODUCTION

Welcome. If you're reading this book, there's a good chance that you want to 'spice things up' in your love life. You and your partner want some new ideas on how to keep the passion going, even though you may have fallen into a rut. Then you have come to the right place.

In the following chapters, this book will teach you new ways to explore your sexuality and sensuality with your partner, how to foster more intimacy between you, and how to enjoy your playtime safely and consensually. It's not just a book that will tell you 'kiss here, grope there, say these words, and boom! You're done.' Hopefully, it will help you be more open with your partner about your desires in the bedroom so that you both can have a more fulfilling sex life. When you change your mentality and see that sex is not just penetration, but also the whole experience, sex becomes more fun and playful. It gives you more room to add new games and to have more fun.

Hopefully, you're reading this together as there will be advice that pertains to everyone. This isn't a book that's just teaching women how to please their men or vice versa. Everything in this book will be geared toward your partnership as a whole.

In the following chapters, you'll read about: opening communication to talk about desires, erogenous zones and how to use them to your advantage, choosing the right toys for your needs and how to include them in your playtime, setting the mood just right for the kind of environment you want to create in the bedroom, all sorts of games you can play with your partner, oral sex and no, it's not just about blowjobs, positions that are going to make sure that everyone is feeling good, and how to carry over the intimacy after the games are done.

Just so we're all on the same page, in this book, the correct terms will be used for the right parts of the body. No euphemisms will be used. The words below will be used with the following definitions:

- Vulva: the exterior of a woman's genitals. This includes the labia, external clitoris, and vaginal opening
- Vagina: the interior canal of a woman's genitals. Not the whole genital area, just the inside.
- Penis: the primary male genital organ
- Scrotum: the pouch that contains a man's testicles

This book will cover a lot and will encourage quite a bit of introspection. You and your partner must keep an open mind while exploring what you both like in the bedroom and approach everything with an open heart. When you keep an open mind, you open yourself up to a more fantastic world of possibilities than you ever thought possible. You'll be able to find more things to try with your partner, and the two of you will feel closer to each other after having opened that line of communication.

CHAPTER 1: COMMUNICATION

Without communication, you can't have good sex. Sure, you can have sex that gets the job done, but without that open line of communication, it'll just be satisfactory when it could be extraordinary. Now, we're not just talking about communicating like, 'yes, I like this' or 'no, I don't like this.' It's about voicing those desires and boundaries even before the clothes come off.

Communication Before Sex

Throughout this book, you'll be met with plenty of suggestions to add to your bedroom playtime. And while you're reading, grab a piece of paper, a notepad, your tablet, whatever you have and create three lists: Want, Will, Won't. A list of items you want to try or feel like you absolutely want to have as part of your sex life, a list of things you are willing to try, but they aren't as pressing or don't feel like necessities, and a list of things you won't do, your hard no boundaries. Both you and your partner should create your own lists. This is about you getting your desires on paper without fear or judgment. You'll share your lists with your partner later.

Ideal items for your WANT list are things you've read about, talked about with your friends, seen on TV or in movies that you really want to try. Thinking about adding this to your sex life makes you want to grab your partner and jump into bed. They should give you a warm feeling when you think about them.

Some items might not seem worth it to put on the list, but some simple actions like 'kissing on the lips, spooning after sex, back rubs, or hugging' should be included. The small things don't need to be left out because they should be a given. Give them the same weight you'd give trying out a new position. Put those small items on your list and talk about them with your partner. Once you put them down on paper, you may realize that you haven't been getting as many small affections you need as you previously thought.

Comparing your Want list with your partner is easy. See where you two have marked down the same items or compatible items. They may have written down that they want to try edging you, and you wrote down that you want to try being edged. Or you both wrote down that you want to try repairman roleplay. You now immediately have some new ideas to bring into the bedroom and can get started.

Items for your WILL list should be things that you've thought about, that intrigue you, and you're willing to give them a try. These items will most likely be things that your partner wants, that you will do, but they might not be your favorite things. You could be willing to give your partner a blow job, but it might not be your favorite thing in the world. Many of your wills might be items that you will do for your partner and their pleasure, even if you don't derive any direct pleasure from them other than making them happy.

Comparing these lists will take a bit more communications than the Want and Won't list. This is a gray area. Talk with your partner about what you like and don't like about the items on your will list. You could be willing to be tied down to the bed during sex if that's something your partner wants to try, but you'd like it to be with a soft material, so it doesn't chafe your skin, and you don't want to be tied down so tightly you can't move. Talk out why you're willing to do it and the circumstances that will make you feel the safest.

If an item is on both of your Will lists, talk about if you even want to do it or if you put it down because you'll do it if it's something your partner wants. Just because you wrote down that you're willing, it doesn't mean you have to do it if neither of you are incredibly interested.

Your Won't list should compile of things you do not want to do. They do not appeal to you. These are your boundaries. It's okay to have something that you don't want to try. Keeping an open mind does not mean that you are open to every possibility. It means you're open to discussing the options outside of your norm. Not every game is going to appeal to every person.

You can populate these lists with anything you consider an intimate act. It could be as simple as: kissing, hugging, hand-holding, etc. Get as many items down into each list as you can. The ideal number would be approximately 30 items per list, but if you can't think of 30 things you are willing to do, just get as many as you can.

It is important to BE HONEST. If you absolutely will not choke your partner during sex, and that's something on their want list, that's something you both need to know so you can talk about it. Communication is key in and out of the bedroom.

More examples of items you can put on your list are: spooning, cooking together as foreplay, massages, being lifted up when you're kissed, hickeys, missionary position, giving and or receiving oral sex, tickling, sensation play, ice, candle wax, anal play, giving or receiving spanks, and everything in between. If something strikes you as intimate or something that could lead to further intimacy, put it on your list.

Remember: items can move from one list to another. You could put fireman roleplay on your will list, and the more you think about it, the more you realize that's something you want to try and want to bring up with your partner, move it over. Alternatively, you could have double penetration on your want list, but then after you try it, you decide that it's not something you ever want to do again; move it over to the won't list. It's okay for your wants and desires to change as well as your boundaries. There are some acts you just won't know you don't like until you try them. As long as you and your partner keep the lines of communication open during your playtime, you have infinite possibilities to explore your sexuality together.

Once you both have your lists and have set aside some time to compare them, see where your similarities and differences lie and write them down on their own list. Chances are there is going to be a little bit of both. If you both have 'use more toys' on your want list, great! Get started with talking about what kinds of toys you would want to include, there will be a whole list of options later on, and start shopping. Maybe you have 'hickeys' on your want list, but your partner has them on their won't list. It's okay to ask them why, but it's important not to pressure them into changing their mind if it's a hard no for them. Maybe they don't want to receive hickeys, but they'd be willing to give you some.

If something is on your won't list, you should never feel pressured to change that if it's something your partner wants. That's why you wrote the lists separately. If it's something you genuinely do not want to do, you don't have to do it. But you can still talk about it. It doesn't mean you have to change your mind, but you might be able to find some common ground that will be something you are both willing to do.

With communicating your wants, wills, and won'ts, it's essential to leave room for a compromise, but you should never compromise on your safety and wellbeing. If your partner has a want that is your won't, and there is no middle ground, you do not have to compromise on your hard boundary.

To explore together, you need to know each other's boundaries. As it stands, you might not know all of your hard no boundaries yet, and that's okay. Now is the time to explore everything remotely exciting and know that you have a way out if something feels too intense, too deep, or doesn't feel good. If you don't like something, you have to have an exit strategy to stop it.

If it's not an enthusiastic 'yes I want to do this' or 'yes, I am willing to give this a try with you within the parameters we have set,' it's a no. When discussing which items from your list to try out, start with your common wants, see how they feel, and decide if they're going to be new permanent additions to your bedroom repertoire. Start slowly. Walk before you run. Don't go from 'missionary all the time' to 'switching positions every 3 seconds.' Most importantly, talk to each other.

Communication During Sex

The most common exit strategy is the use of a safe word. A safe word can be a word or phrase, although it's recommended not to be longer than a couple of words, that would not naturally come up in any form of playtime. Common safewords are cities, relative's names, or foods. Make it something personal to you and your partner that you both will easily be able to remember.

Another common exit strategy is the color system: red, yellow, green. When the person who is guiding the action adds something new to your playtime, such as tying the other up or changing the rhythm you're going in, it's essential to check in with your partner by simply asking 'what's your color?' If your partner responds 'red,' that means you stop all action and reassess, figure out what they don't like and how you can make them feel better. If they say 'yellow,' you can keep going, but proceed with caution. Slow down, ask them if something is hurting them or what you can change to help them feel safe. If they respond 'green,' keep ongoing.

Additionally, the color system can easily be used as a regular safe word. Instead of saying 'apple' or 'Tallahassee,' if something doesn't feel right and you want to stop, just say 'red,' and that will be your partner's cue to stop what they're doing, or 'yellow' and they will slow down. You can both decide what can be changed so you can both feel comfortable and safe in your intimate time.

Talk about what you or your partner saying red means before you even take your clothes off. It's not a bad thing for either of you to feel the need to say it; it's just the opposite. By voicing your feelings when something feels off, you're communicating your desires as well as your dislikes. Neither of you should feel ashamed or guilty for having said it or caused the other to say it. It's entirely natural not to know how something will affect you until you are in the middle of the situation. You tried, it didn't work out as you planned, so you're taking a step back to figure out how you can make it better. It shows a great deal of trust in your partner that you're stopping the scenario so you each can make it better for the both of you.

Even if you don't think you need a safe word or a color system, it's still incredibly important to communicate during sex. The occasional 'is this okay?' can mean a world of difference. Your partner might not have said something otherwise if you didn't ask. Using the color system in all kinds of play is a great way to keep those lines of communication open.

Pay attention to each other's body language and facial expressions. What's coming out of your partner's mouth might contradict how they hold their head or body. They could be telling you to keep going, but their arms are lying flat against the bed, and they're looking at the ceiling like they'd rather be anywhere else.

Look for non-verbal signs of encouragement: hands gripping at your shoulders or back, moving your hips along with your partner. If they can't keep their hands off of you, assuming they aren't tied down to something, that's a good sign that they are enjoying themselves.

Communication After Sex

Communication after sex is just as important as during and before. It helps you both decompress and talk about what you liked, what you maybe didn't like, and what you want to try again. After trying a new toy for the first time, you may discover that you didn't like how it felt, and you don't want to use it again. Tell your partner! They might have loved it and assumed you did too unless you told them otherwise. It can't be stressed enough; talk it out.

Maybe you didn't like where the vibrator was placed, perhaps it was on too high, or maybe it was uncomfortable to hold. Talk it out with your partner and see if there is a middle ground you two can find or if your new toy needs to be shelved.

It is especially important to talk after something goes wrong, one of you needed to stop because something was painful, uncomfortable, or too intense, or something doesn't sit right with you now that you're done. If anything your partner is doing is less than satisfactory, tell them, reassure them that you love them, and you just want to make your sex better for both of you.

Pillow talk does not need to be awkward. It can be sweet and genuine, telling each other how much you love what you just did together, how much closer you feel, and how much you want to do it again. Communication isn't just about telling each other what you didn't like, while that is a big part of it. It's also about expressing the good in your sex life and encouraging each other to keep exploring new games and toys to add to your sex life.

Your talk can be as explicit as 'using sex dice to get in the mood was a good idea. We should do that again next time.' Or it can be a simple as cuddling up with your partner and whispering in their ear, 'I loved that so much.' It's important to be direct and clear about what you liked about the sex you had so your partner is encouraged, and you can keep exploring.

Go back over your Want, Will, and Won't list after you've tried out some of the items. See if there's anything you want to move around. Tickling was previously on your Will list, but the way your partner tickled your sides while they kissed you felt amazing, and you want to do it again, move it to your Want. You thought you wanted to try being spanked, but it didn't do anything for you, move it to your Will or Won't, depending on how much you disliked it. Do this together with your partner so you both know where you stand and with what you can move forward.

CHAPTER 2: EROGENOUS ZONES AND FOREPLAY

What are the Erogenous Zones?

Erogenous zones are essential to turning on your partner. Coming from the Greek' eros,' which is a type of love, and 'genous' or producing, stimulating the erogenous zones get us in the mood. Erogenous zones don't just mean your genitals, although touching them does help. Simply put, they are the areas of our body that get us hot and bothered. And they are your key to getting your partner turned on well before you've entered the bedroom.

Everyone is going to have different parts of their body that gets them going. What may have worked for your last partner might not work for your current one. But most people will enjoy stimulation in some of the same set of erogenous zones: the scalp, the ears, the neck, the inner forearm, the inner wrist, the stomach, the base of the spine, the butt, the inner thighs, and behind the knees.

Keep in mind, some of these might not seem like the most sensitive areas of your body, but during sex, or just after, your nerves are on fire, everything is extra sensitive. You previously didn't think the inside of your wrist could be sexy suddenly makes you feel all tingly when your partner kisses you there when you caress their cheek.

You might not think your stomach is very sensitive until your partner tickles over it lightly with their fingers or a piece of fabric. Suddenly having them touch you there makes you squirm and want more touch and affection. Ears don't seem sexy to you until your partner sneaks up behind you and blows gently against the back of your ear. The only way to find out if these areas of your body work for you is to test them out and see.

These areas of the body are erogenous zones either because of their inherent sensitivity or because of their proximity to the genital nerves. Some zones, like the ears and the neck, are body parts that get us hot and bothered because they have hundreds of nerve endings compacted into small spaces, thus increasing their sensitivity. In other cases, like the inner thighs and butt, the nerves stimulated by touching them are closely related to the nerves in the genitals.

Not everyone is going to experience pleasure and sensitivity from all of these zones. Some people may experience nothing in all of these. That's why it's important to explore your body with your partner. Much like how every person finds different body parts on others sexy, we find different parts of our bodies sexy. You might really like having your palm kissed. It drives you wild. In comparison, your partner might feel nothing when you kiss their palm. Every body is different.

Why is Foreplay Important?
Starting the mood before you get down to business is very important. It not only primes you to have a good time, but it also makes you that much more aroused when you do get going with penetrative sex. Foreplay is not just a precursor to sex. Foreplay is sex. It makes sex better. Not every sexual encounter has a primary sex act to signal the beginning and completion of sex.

Foreplay and teasing can be the whole experience with some penetration added into the mix.

With foreplay, there is no beginning, middle, and end. It's all one big experience. You end when you decide you're done with playtime. A survey conducted by Glamour found that on average, couples were spending 5-9 minutes on foreplay, with 33% of participants reporting that. In contrast, only 8% of participants reported spending 20 minutes or more on foreplay. That average can change. You can change your average.

When you change your definition of foreplay, you realize that it lasts much longer than you thought. Anything that turns you on and increases the intimacy with your partner is foreplay. It's not just making out while you get your clothes off. Foreplay extends the intimacy and arousal, in and out of the bedroom. If you and your partner cook dinner together, that can be considered foreplay. If you watch a movie, cuddled up together under the blankets, gently stroking each other's arms, that's foreplay. It can be anything that gets you and your partner in the mood, and keeps you in the mood, for intimacy. It's not just a little bit of oral sex and make outs before the main event. The whole thing is the main event.

Foreplay is healthy for you, not just for your sex life. Increased time spent on foreplay increases the build-up of oxytocin or the love hormone. Your body releases this during foreplay, sex, and in the aftercare spent in your partner's arms. It's a natural pain reliever. And it helps you feel closer to your partner.

If you've completed your Want, Will, and Won't lists you should have several ways to get started with foreplay, but if not, there are some suggestions below to get you started, and you can add them to your list if they entice you.

How to Incorporate Erogenous Zones into your Foreplay
Start with a little erogenous zone exploration.

Lie down on your back. Going head to toe, start with your scalp. Have your partner run their fingers through your hair, scratch their nails against your scalp. Does it feel good? Does it leave you tingling and wanting to pull them closer to you? If it does, you've found an erogenous zone. Keep going.

Maybe now your partner brings their lips into play, and they start to nibble on your earlobe. Notice how it makes you feel. For some people, their ears don't feel much of anything. And that's okay. Let your partner move to your neck, kissing all over it. Let your partner know how you're feeling. Give them verbal and non-verbal cues. If you want them to keep going, tell them too. Lean into their touch. If you don't like it, tell them, and they can continue with their path.

Your inner forearm might be more sensitive to lips or light fabrics than just a simple touch. Try holding your arms up above your head and have your partner run some material, like a tie or the edge of a scarf, over your inner arm. Let them kiss the inside of your wrist as you caress their cheek. If it doesn't make you feel much, it's okay. You might feel more once you're more turned on. You can always revisit this zone later.

Let your partner do the same over your stomach. They can gently kiss it, maybe paying particular attention to your navel or the area where your abdomen meets your hips. They can tease it with the tie or scarf, or just tickle you if that's something you both are willing to try. Now turn onto your stomach.

Have your partner run their fingers along your back, stopping before they get to your butt. Just let them focus on the base of the spine. Right there is a shield-shaped bone called the sacrum. The sacral nerve, located at the bottom of the spine, is connected to your genitals' nerves. For some people, being massaged here can feel very similar to being touched directly on your genitals.

Next, let them move down to your butt. Your partner is not going anywhere near your anus or trying to penetrate you. They're just going to massage the muscle, squeeze it and release tension. They can run their fingers along you lightly, scratch their nails against the soft skin like they did with your scalp. If you've decided spanking is something you would want to try, they could start with light taps and slowly build up to harder spanks. Spread out the spanks, don't focus on one area for too long. Once your skin starts to turn pink, it's time to spread the love to another site.

From here, your partner can spread your legs a little bit and run their fingers along your inner thighs. They should be getting close to your genitals, but not touch them. They're still finding your erogenous zones. Like before, they can use their fingers, their lips, their tongue, or some light fabric to see just how sensitive you are there.

They can keep going down the backs of your legs to see if you're just as sensitive behind your knees. You might not be; you might love it. You won't know until you try.

This kind of exploration of erogenous zones is excellent to try once you're in the bedroom and already in the mood. Once you know your erogenous zones, there are great ways to incorporate touching them and stimulating them before you've even gotten each other's clothes off.

Foreplay Outside of the Bedroom
As stated earlier in this chapter, foreplay isn't just the opening act to the headliner, foreplay is a leading lady, and it deserves to be treated as such. You can start foreplay well before you plan to enter the bedroom. And you and your partner can use the erogenous zones you've discovered on yourselves to your advantage.

Start the foreplay once you both come home from work, if it's a weeknight, or you're in for the evening on the weekend. Cook dinner together. Don't make anything too heavy or extravagant. A full stomach doesn't mix well with bedroom intimacy. Whatever you do make, prepare it together. Don't go all Ghost and have one person behind the other, guiding their hands as they chop vegetables. But one of you can be cooking while the other is prepping more ingredients. Or one can make the entree while the other makes the side dish. Take the time you might otherwise be separate and spend it together.

While you're chopping vegetables for the salad, your partner could come up and wrap their arms around you from behind, laying their hands on your stomach or your hips. They could rest their chin on your shoulder, kiss your neck or behind your ear. Let them play with your erogenous zones while you're cooking.

If your kitchen or dining room allows it, sit beside one another or on adjacent sides of the table, not across from each other. Sit as close to each other as possible without getting in the way of eating. If you can, rest your leg against your partner's to keep that physical contact as you're eating. Much like the fatty foods, go easy on the wine or other alcohol. You'll want a clear head if you're planning to introduce new games or toys tonight.

Watch a movie or an episode of a show you both like together. Keep the anticipation building before you start. The longer you go before you jump into bed, the better it's going to be. Curl up on the couch together and tangle your legs together or spoon on the couch if it's big enough. All of this will foster intimacy and extend it to every corner of your home, not just your bed.

If you don't want to make a night of it, but you want to jump-start your brain into relaxation and intimacy, try a massage. You don't have to strip down and get all kinds of scented oils. You can give or receive a massage with all of your clothes on your body.

Lie down on your bed on your stomach, prop up your head, so you're comfortable, and let your partner pamper you. Tell them if you're having any aches or pains that they could focus on massaging out and enjoy the feeling of their hands on your body. If you're the one giving the massage, move in slow, deep motions, pay attention if your partner tenses or winces. Make sure you're not causing them any pain. The idea is just to get them as relaxed as possible.

It's tempting to massage their butt; it's right there in front of you. Unless your partner has told you they are having pain back there, avoid it for now. The idea is to relax their muscles and increase sensitivity all over. Turn their entire body into one big erogenous zone. Massage down their legs and feet if they've been walking around and standing all day. If they've been sitting at a desk, focus on their upper back and shoulders, maybe moving down their arms every few strokes. Listen to what their body is telling you. If they move into your touch, keep going. If you get no response, ask them if they'd like you to massage a different spot and move on.

Ask your partner how they feel, if there are any areas you missed that feel very tense, or if they need a moment before you start to try and take their clothes off. Massages are incredibly relaxing, and some people need a few minutes to get themselves out of that relaxed floppy state.

Make your whole living space your play space. It's important to keep an open mind when trying new positions and games. It's also important to keep an open mind about where you explore your playtime. If your couch is comfortable or the floor of your living room has a cozy rug, try fooling around or giving your partner a massage in there. Turn every available space in your home into an opportunity for foreplay and intimacy.

If you choose to do this, make sure you're as comfortable as possible. Add pillows if you're playing on a hard surface or around you as a buffer if you're giving the couch a try, and you're afraid of falling off. Make sure the blinds and curtains are closed if you're worried about neighbors seeing you. Even if you're not concerned with neighbors seeing you and you just want that extra security, close your blinds. If you are playing anywhere near an open window and your home overlooks a busy street, someone will be able to see you. If that's what you're into, then it's no trouble. But if you're not ready to try exhibitionism, or showing off, just yet, close your blinds and have fun.

Foreplay Inside of the Bedroom

If the clothes are already starting to come off and you want to get going, you can give them a massage once you're both naked or stripped down to your underwear. When you're giving a massage skin to skin, you should use some kind of lubricants like baby oil or massage oil to make sure you aren't chafing your partner's skin too severely. Use a scent that you both find calming and relaxing like lavender or eucalyptus. It should be something you both enjoy. If the smell is powerful, just make sure to wash your hands before you start to touch each other more intimately. Some of those fragrances don't mix well with the sensitive skin of your genitals.

Sit on your partner's hips as carefully as you can without hurting them and run your fingers up and down their back, just along their spine. Let the oils heat up against your hand and their skin. Don't be afraid to put some pressure on if that's what your partner wants.

If your partner likes to feel more pressure as you massage them, you can put more of your body weight on them. Rock your hips a little as you massage their back, sides, and arms. Make them as relaxed as possible.

Much like before, when you were exploring each other's erogenous zones, get as close to each other's genitals as you can. Touch your partner's thighs, hips, butt, stomach, anywhere you can think. Just keep teasing your fingers closer and closer until our partner is begging for more contact.

Draw small circles with your fingertips, draw big circles with your whole hand. See what your partner likes and how they react to the touch. For some people, they will simply be too ticklish for this kind of stimulation. Some people like being tickled. Talk to each other and check-in with a simple 'does this feel good?' any time you're trying something new. Keep those lines of communication as open as possible.

When you're at the point where you can't possibly stand the teasing anymore, but you don't want to go right to penetrative sex, move on to other forms of touching: oral sex and use of your hands. If you've felt in the past that oral sex doesn't feel as good as 'normal' sex, give it a try after you've spent some time teasing one another. Now that you're all sensitive and tingly, it could feel entirely different.

Ladies: Don't worry about how your vulva tastes or smells. Unless you have some sort of yeast infection, you're going to taste good. Do not use any perfumes or scented lotions to make it taste differently. It's going to taste like a vulva.

Keep teasing each other, even after you've established that you're beginning oral sex. Move your lips slowly toward your partner's vulva or penis. Use your tongue to draw the same shapes you'd just been drawing with your fingers. Take your time building up to that perfect moment where you finally come in contact with the part of their body your partner has wanted you to touch the most all night. It's worth the wait.

Foreplay should not be thrown to the wayside. Sure, you can have entirely pleasurable quickies with no preamble. But think about the quickies you've had in the past. Were you or your partner doing something to get the other turned on before you got the other alone? Did they keep bumping into you, brushing their hand against your hip? That's foreplay. The only definition of foreplay is that it comes before you play. But it's not a specific subset of activities. Your entire relationship could be foreplay if you try hard enough. Foreplay is only dull and restrictive when we close our minds to the notion that anything other than penetrative sex isn't sex. It's all part of the intimate experience you have with your partner. How you categorize it all is up to you.

CHAPTER 3: TOYS

Toys are not just for kids. While most people assume sex toys are a modern invention, artifacts dug up by archeologists were dated back to Ancient Greece that historians believe to be homemade dildos. In the mid to late 1800s, doctors invented vibrators to use on patients diagnosed with 'hysteria,' a common diagnosis for women exhibiting irritability, shortness of breath, insomnia, and sexual desire. The cure was an orgasm, and doctors were getting tired of using their hands.

But sex toys are much more than just for female masturbation. Many toys in the current market are geared toward couples to use together. Many are even designed specifically for men. In this chapter, we're going to go over all of them, they're uses, and how they can be used to better your playtime.

How To Decide Which Toy is Right for You

First and foremost, shop for your toys together. If there is a sex shop nearby and you feel comfortable going there, go together and look at toys together. Get a feel for the different sizes, shapes, weights, and types. There will be someone who can help you decide what kind of toy will work best for your wants and needs.

Additionally, the employee can make sure that any add ons you would need for the toy, such as lube or cleanser, will be compatible with your toy. Not every lube is right for every toy, and you shouldn't clean every toy the same way. Do not use a silicone-based lubricant with a silicone toy. Putting silicone lube on a silicone toy will cause the toy to deteriorate. The employees are there to answer your questions and make sure you are happy with your purchase when you leave the store.

If you don't have a store nearby or are not quite ready to go out in public and buy a sex toy, there are plenty of online retailers who ship in discreet packaging so that no one knows that large brown parcel is a box full of fun. Simply do a web search for 'online sex toy retailer,' You can find some list articles with great selections of websites to choose from.

Most online retailers will split up their toys by categories, like below, for men and women, and then subcategories underneath. You can read reviews, see the technical specs, materials, waterproofness, and get recommendations on products to use with it.

No matter the toy you choose to add to your playtime or the method you choose to shop, make the decision together. It's nice to be able to surprise your partner every once in a while. But when you're first starting, you need to be comfortable talking with them about what you want and need out of a new toy.

Toys for Women
Vibrators. Not every vibrator is a dildo, and not every dildo vibrates. Vibrators come in all shapes and sizes and can be added easily into any position or scenario. We'll go over each kind from biggest to smallest, starting with wand vibrators.

One of the most iconic, the wand vibrator, is perfect for couples to use together. Its trademark is a long handle with a bulbous end that you hold against your clit. For women who like stimulation over a wide area, this is perfect. Your partner can easily control it while they are penetrating you. These vibrators lead very well to scenarios involving bondage because of their handle. The toy is easily tied to your leg, so you can't move it or away from it. Or your partner could tease you with it by sitting behind you, or far away from you, and hold the toy against your vulva, not letting you touch them while they manipulate the toy. It's a great toy to use for edging.

Be warned. These toys can be very powerful because an electrical cord often powers them. You may want to visit a sex shop if you have one nearby, see the toy firsthand, and feel how powerful it is. Some women find these toys too powerful, and they don't get any pleasure from them. That's completely normal. If you can't get to a store to see one in person, opt for a rechargeable or battery operated toy. They usually are not as powerful because of their built-in power supply.

Another equally as recognizable vibrator is the rabbit vibrator. Its shape distinguishes this toy. It usually will have dildo shaped end with an attachment coming off of the side that looks like bunny ears, hence the name, to tease your clit at the same time. You can find rabbits with a wide variety of settings and features. Some only have vibration through the rabbit ears; some have vibration through the ears and insertable. Sometimes the insertable section creates a thrusting motion; the possibilities are endless.

Rabbit vibrators are great for solo play, help you get warmed up, or be used together during foreplay. A little mutual masturbation never hurt anyone in the bedroom. You get to set the pace, the speed of the toy, and show off to your partner that you're having a perfect time. Or you can let your partner take charge and hold the toy.

Insertable vibrators can look very much like dildos or other toys, and they fall into that gray area of some vibrators are dildos but dildos are not necessarily vibrators. G-spot vibrators are another common name for insertable vibrators. They are generally known for their long curved shape, sometimes with a bulb at the end. But there can be insertable vibrators that are long and pointed, short and pointed, or anything in between. In truth, any toy is insertable, unless the packaging says explicitly 'for external use only.

The smallest vibrators still pack a punch. Most commonly, they are known as bullet vibrators because of their shape. They are small, pill, or bullet-shaped devices that fit in the palm of your hand. They are great to have your partner use against your clit, or for you to use against yourself while giving your partner oral sex. They are tiny, discreet, and often very quiet.

These are great to use as part of foreplay, for mutual masturbation, or during penetrative sex. What's great about these toys is that they come in all kinds of shapes and sizes. The bigger ones are better to keep at home, but the smaller ones can fit in a purse or carry on bag and easily be taken with you on a trip anywhere.

Finger style vibrators are another type or bullet vibrator. Despite the name, these are not vibrators that look like fingers, but they fit on your finger. Usually, these toys are bullet style vibrators, maybe a little bit smaller, that going into a sleeve that fits on your finger. So you or your partner can turn your finger into a vibrator.

Usually, these toys will have some texture on the rubber covering the vibrator to add extra sensations to your clit and vulva. These toys are small but well designed. They are powerful. Go easy with them and learn what feels right. You may like them on your clit by themselves, or with some internal stimulation via your partner. You might like them internally. But make sure you check the technical specs on your toy to make sure it is approved for internal use. Not every toy can. You don't want to break your toy mid-session and ruin the mood.

Finger vibrators are great to use during penetrative sex. Since they are no bigger than your finger, they don't get in the way and fit anywhere your hand does.

Butterfly vibrator is in a class all its own. The beauty of most sex toys is the name is very descriptive. Butterfly vibrators are just that, vibrators that often look like butterflies. Traditionally, butterfly vibrators have three qualifications: they are insertable, they are wearable, and they cover the whole vulva. Many of them have butterfly-like designs. The head leans against the clit, and wings vibrating against your labia and the rest of the vulva.

Most importantly, these toys are wearable. Butterfly vibrators not only vibrate your entire vulva, but they also stay in place because of the dildo attached to the 'body' of the butterfly. You slide this end inside of you until the outer portion of the toy is flush against your vulva, then you turn it on.

A remote control controls most models of butterfly vibrators you're going to find. Some will have a cord connecting the controller to the toy, and others will have a completely wireless remote, so your partner doesn't even have to be anywhere near you to stimulate you.

These are great to tease. Often the shaft of the toy and the body of the butterfly function completely separately so your partner can tease your g-spot, then your clit, then both, never letting you get used to the same sensation for long.

Toys like this would be great to be used in tandem with some form of bondage play and edging, more on that in a later chapter. Your partner could tie your hands up so you can't remove the toy, or connect your feet to the legs of the bed so you can't close them, and do what they want with you. If you're still having trouble reaching orgasm, toys like these are great to get used to internal and clitoral stimulation at the same time.

Dildos and Insertable. Dildos, much like vibrators, come in all shapes and sizes. The most important things to consider when it comes to insertable toys are the material. You don't want to purchase anything that will be harmful to your body or hard to clean. Porous materials like jelly toys or phthalates are going to tick off both of those boxes. If you already have a toy made of the soft jelly material you don't want to part with, it may be worth putting a condom on it going forward. If any toy you own contains phthalates, throw it away. The material is a carcinogen and linked to causing cancer. The risk doesn't outweigh any benefits. If you're buying new toys, look for dildos made of silicone, glass, ABS plastic, metal, and other non-porous materials. They're much safer, with little to no risk to your body, and very easy to clean. Just a little soap and water and you're good to go.

Think about the feeling you want from the toy. If you want it to feel more lifelike, then go for softer material like silicone. If you're going to add in some sensation or temperature play, consider a glass or metal toy that you can chill before bringing it into the bedroom.

For some added fun, if you're interested in sex toy science experiments, there are kits that you can buy to make your own dildo shaped like your partner's penis. When it comes to dildos, the sky is the limit when you look at sizes, shapes, and colors, so why not have one that feels familiar?

You and your partner can use dildos together; they can watch you use it on yourself, or use it for some double penetration either during penetrative sex or while you are performing oral sex. The possibilities only end with your imagination.

Another popular insertable toy is vaginal balls, also known as Kegel balls. These are a set of two balls connected with a long retrieval cord coming off the end. You use them by inserting them into the vagina. Each ball has a small weight that will roll around inside. As they fall to the bottom due to gravity, the vaginal muscles will sense that whatever is inside is falling out and contract in an attempt to keep the object inside. These are great to use before having sex to help strengthen your pelvic floor muscles. Put them in before date night begins for a surprise for your partner, or put them in together as you start your foreplay.

If you're interested in anal play, butt plugs might be something you want to look at. Anything you are inserting into your anus needs to have a flared base or some kind of retrieval cord to ensure it doesn't get lost inside of you. The rectum is not like the vagina. Your vagina is more like a pocket; there's only so much space for the toy to go.

If a toy does get pulled into your rectum and you can't retrieve it, please visit the emergency room immediately.

The anal toys' material is particularly important as there is more harmful bacterial inside the anal cavity. Many anal toys consist of metal and plastic for this reason. They are non-porous, easy to clean, and in many cases, they are dishwasher safe, so you don't have to worry about that bacteria sticking around.

Extra Anal Toy Safety Tip: It's okay for you to use a toy vaginally and then anally, but not the other way around. The bacteria mentioned above do not mix well with the ph balance of the vagina. Once a toy has been used for anal play, it needs to remain an anal play toy until you properly sanitize it.

Other Toys that Vibrate. Another popular toy that doesn't quite qualify as a vibrator is the air pulsation stimulator. They are toys with a little opening designed to go around the clitoris and simulate oral sex. Most come with various speeds from very soft to very hard, and work to simulate a mouth sucking on your clit. These are great to use during foreplay or with your partner deciding how high the toy will go.

Many toy companies make vibrators designed for you to wear them during penetrative sex. These toys often have 'we' in the name somewhere and have a pincer-like shape. Their design allows for one half of the toy to be inserted and rest against the g-sport, while the other half curves up the vulva's front to vibrate against the clit. During penetrative sex, your partner will be able to feel the vibration against his penis, and the thrusting motion will often press the inserted half of the toy harder against your g-spot.

Other toys. If you have a lack of sensitivity in your breasts and nipples, some toys help with that. Nipple clamps and nipple suckers will put pressure or tension on the nipples and surrounding areola.

Traditionally, nipple clamps are for BDSM play, but you can use them if you enjoy a little pain with your pleasure and would like prolonged pressure during your playtime. These are usually a set of two small metal clamps, sometimes attached by a chain so that your partner can tug on them. Store-bought clamps will usually have a way to adjust the tension so that you can find the pressure that feels perfect to you.

If you want to see if this sort of nipple play is for you, you can give this sort of sensation a try with clothespins. Just be very careful and don't leave them on for too long. Build up to having them on for more extended periods while you're getting used to them

Nipple suckers are like nipple clamps in that they allow for prolonged pressure on your nipple. You can get these in various sizes, so they go over just the nipple itself or around the surrounding areola as well. These come in matching pairs or sets of different sizes. They work like a suction cup, as the name would suggest. You place the cup end over your nipple and use the plunger or the squeeze end to create suction over your nipple, letting the skin get sucked in. Some people find this alone to be incredibly pleasurable on its own. The increase of blood flow to the area will increase sensitivity. Others find the release of the suction to be satisfying as well. As with most other toys, go slowly, communicate with your partner, and pull back if something becomes too painful. It's all right to like a little pain with your pleasure. But it's okay if there comes a point when there's too much pain. Say yellow or red, reassess, and have fun.

Toys for Men
Strokers, or male masturbators, or sleeves are very useful in foreplay. Handjobs are nice, but sometimes it could be fun to add a little more to that sort of teasing. These toys are usually some sort of rubber or silicone sleeve inside of a rigid housing, so it's more comfortable to hold. The sleeves are made of a material meant to mimic the human body and come in all kinds of shapes, sizes, and colors.

Manufacturers design the toys to look like body parts, mouths, butts, vaginas, or they could just look like a round opening. The interior will often have bumps and ridges to add extra stimulation to the shaft of the penis. Simply add a little lubrication, and you're good to go.

You can use some strokers without an outer casing. These allow you to use your hand to mold them better against the penis.

There's no difference or benefit to one or the other. With a toy that comes in an outer shell, the shell decides the tightness of the sleeve. With a toy that has no outer shell, your hand determines the tightness. It's all up to personal preference.

These toys are great to use during mutual masturbation. If one partner is using a toy, the other should get to have one too, right? Get into a comfortable position and masturbate, as usual, only this time it'll be with the toy instead of your hand.

These are also useful for edging. Because you're using the toy, and not your whole body, it's much easier to work your partner up slowly and ease them back down again.

Cock rings can be extremely pleasurable for men and women. Their primary function is to restrict blood flow to the penis, allowing men to have longer, harder erections. Traditionally, they are stretchy rings of silicone that can go up against the base of the penis, behind the scrotum and sitting flush against a man's pelvis, or they go just around your scrotum.

Because their primary function is to tighten and constrict, you need to use them safely. Use lubricant to make sure the rubber or silicone doesn't irritate your skin as you slide it over the head of your penis and down into position. Slide the ring over a flaccid or semi-erect penis. If you are experiencing a full erection, the ring will likely be too tight, and you won't be able to get it fixed properly.

Once the ring is in place, blood can flow in, but it cannot flow out. This restriction results in a more prolonged and sometimes harder erection. As this is the primary function, do not leave this on for too long. The general guideline is that you should not wear one for longer than 20 to 30 minutes. If you're starting, it's always better to start low and work your way up to wearing it for longer.

Start with a basic ring made of silicone and see if you like the feeling it gives you. Eventually, you can work your way up to cock rings that vibrate. The vibration will allow for extra stimulation for both of you during penetrative sex.

Toys for Couples

Many sex toys marketed as 'toys for couples' lean towards exploration in BDSM play. Whips, floggers, handcuffs, sex swings, oh my! There are so many options and so many places to start. More so than the list above, it's essential to purchase these toys together. Once you've developed a rhythm and know more about each other's likes, you can buy toys to surprise the other. But if the toy is for both of you, you should buy it together to make sure it meets everyone's needs.

Sex swings are a trendy place to start when looking to add something extra to your bedroom time. Despite the name, most sex swings don't operate like playground swings. You can buy a free-standing apparatus to house the swing, or one that you can hang from the ceiling, so you have the full range of motion, but most that are commercially available are hung off of a door.

These models have a counterweight that you hang over the top of your door and close it to lock it into place. They have a seat for you or your partner to rest in with handles and stirrups to make sure no one feels like they're going to fall off. With these swings, your partner can carefully swing you towards them, so you don't swing back and hit the door, and you can enjoy a feeling of weightlessness.

Couples toys kits are very popular. Most sex toy retailers sell kits that let you try a variety of toys together for one price. Some kits are different sizes of dildos or anal toys, and others are kits with items to try out various kinky toys. If you and your partner are interested in trying any aspect of BDSM, these kits are a great place to start because they are cheap, made for comfort, and you'll get the general idea of the basics of BDSM without having to buy a lot of different items.

Basic kinky kits will usually come with a blindfold, a set of handcuffs or restraints, and something to aid in sensation play (a flogger or something to tickle and tease you with). The handcuffs and bonds are soft and won't hurt or chafe due to prolonged exposure. But it's essential to test them out before you cuff yourself to the bed. Restraints will have different tightnesses, so try out the bonds without attaching them to anything to find the level that makes you feel secure but not trapped. It should be snug but not so tight you lose circulation to your hands.

The most common toy used for sensation play is called a flogger. These are straps of fabric bunched together at a handle. They can be used for light sensation play, gently running the material up and down your body. Or more formidable sensation play, by smacking the whole bunch against your partner at once. Do this with caution, and not over susceptible areas of the body. Lightly tap the fabric against your breasts, butt, or inner thighs. Avoid slapping the flogger against your stomach, as this can be extremely painful. Communicate with your partner. If you feel like you can take more, encourage them by asking for more, harder, another. If it's too hard, ask them to slow down or, if you're using the color system, say yellow. Work together to find what feels right. Pain can be pleasurable when administered correctly and only when everything is safe and consensual.

Sex furniture is a category most don't even think about. There are pillows and props designed to help you make your bedroom time as pleasurable and comfortable as possible. Usually, there's a waterproof or machine washable material over the top, so you never have to worry about getting them too dirty. They come in all shapes and sizes. Some are wedge-shaped to lift your hips or your back, some are heart-shaped, and some even have slots and pockets to add your favorite toys.

Whichever toy you choose, make that first decision together and keep exploring. When you add toys to your sex life, the possibilities are endless.

CHAPTER 4: THE FEMALE ORGASM

At first glance, one might think there is no difference between the male and female orgasm. In truth, both are simply the quick release of muscular tension at the peak of sexual arousal. Pelvic floor muscles contract, blood rushes to the genital region, and we are overcome with a pleasurable sensation that keeps us coming back for more. If it didn't feel good, we wouldn't do it.

Despite the similarities, how men and women achieve orgasm is vastly different. It's a very straight forward path for men: manipulation of the penis very often leads to orgasm. But for women, the course is not as linear. Every woman is different.

The female orgasm has one function: to bring pleasure. Because of how the body works, men release a peptide called somatostatin that reduces sexual arousal after ejaculation. They orgasm, ejaculate, the body tells them 'okay, you have done your reproductive duty' and they're done. Women don't do that. Their refractory period, the time after orgasm before one can start stimulation again, is much shorter than men. And in some cases, it's entirely non-existent. Once they've gotten started, many women can keep orgasming one right after the other without stopping.

One common misconception is that the penis and vagina were initially the same organs. As development in the womb begins, the theory goes that the original organ forms into one or the other. But in reality, the clitoris is the female equivalent of the penis. It has a head covered by a protective hood, internally legs are protruding, and two bulb-like glands, known as the crura and vestibular bulbs, respectively, much like the vas deferens and testicles. The clitoris, or clit as it will be known going forward, is far more than meets the eye. The clit is vital for female pleasure. It's the only function is to bring about orgasm.

Another common misconception is that there can be a clitoral orgasm and a vaginal orgasm. When in fact, an orgasm achieved without direct stimulation to the clitoral head, the clit is still the cause; it's just much more extensive than we initially thought. The internal clit can easily be accessed by stimulating the vulva around the vaginal opening either with a toy, fingers, mouth, grinding, and internally through penetration.

If you're unsure if you've ever had an orgasm, chances are you haven't. The female orgasm only seems mysterious because women are taught not to learn about their bodies and explore what feels right. But we're going to fix that today. If you've had one, you'd know it. They're hard to miss. The more you know about your own anatomy, the better you can teach your partner how to pleasure you and get you that big O.

Here Are a Few Tips to Help You Reach Orgasm
1. Masturbate. If you don't know your body, you can't expect someone else to understand it better. Touch yourself, explore your vulva with your fingers, grab a mirror, and take a look at it. Find your clit. Try different ways of touching it. Some women like slow and steady strokes, some women like fast strokes. Some women like circles, some women like up and down. Try it all and see what works well for you.

Learn everything you can about your own body. You need to know all that there is to know before you can expect someone else to be able to give you pleasure.

Don't just focus on your vulva. Touch all over your body and see how it feels when you touch your breasts or your nipples. Learn how every touch makes your body feel. If you have smaller breasts, you're likely to be more sensitive there. If you have larger breasts, you will experience lessened sensitivity there, but you might have higher sensitivity down your stomach or along your inner thighs. Take the time to learn every inch of your body.

Get yourself as aroused as possible before you touch your vulva. Watch porn, read erotica, look at a picture of your partner. Use anything that will get you in the mood and turned on.

Once you've gotten yourself aroused, move your hand between your legs, and touch everywhere but your clit. It's tempting for that to be the first place you go, but if you wait just a little longer, it's going to feel even better. Touch your labia, tease your vaginal entrance, or even run your hands up and down your inner thighs. Get as close to your clit as you can without touching it.

When it feels like you might explode if you don't touch yourself soon, that's when you start to brush your clit. Start slowly and softly, building up speed and pressure if you need it. You might, and you might not. Right now, it's all about learning what your body likes. Find out if you can touch your clit directly or if that's too sensitive. You might need to keep your fingers on top of your clitoral hood. You might like stimulation to your internal clit, and thus you'll need to use your hand to rub over your entire vulva to get to it.

Once you've figured out the rhythm and movement that feels good, keep going. Get yourself as close to that peak as you can, then ease back, then get yourself to just before the precipice again, and reduce back again. Repeat that cycle a couple of times until you get right to that peak and you can't ease back, keep going. Don't stop. You'll know you're close when you feel the cramp in your arm, but you still can't stop.

2. Use toys to make it a little bit easier. If you've tried using your hands to masturbate, or you've tried using your masturbation techniques with your partner, and nothing is working, it's okay to introduce toys into the mix. Lots of women achieve their first orgasm through the help of toys. If you don't know which to buy, go back to the last chapter and look through the list provided. Discuss with your partner what you want the toy to do and if you'll be using this by yourself or with them.

If you're going to get a toy just for yourself, start small and cheap to figure out what you like. It's not worth spending a lot of money on a toy that you don't like. Start with a small bullet vibrator or an insertable vibrator that you can use externally or internally. You're trying to learn about your body; it's okay to need the right tools.

3. Don't focus on having an orgasm. Whether it's with your partner or on your own, the more you focus on that end goal, the further from you it's going to see. Focus on your body, how you feel, what feels good and what doesn't. Neither sex nor

masturbation has to result in orgasm. They can just be about enjoying the sensations and feeling close to your partner. But if an orgasm is something you'd like to achieve, the more you fixate on it, the further from you it's going to be.

4. Tease yourself. Don't just focus on your clit and your vagina. If you have sensitive breasts or nipples, try spending more time focusing on them. Run your fingers, or your partner's fingers, along the sides, tops, underneath the breasts. Use different pressures and sensations. On one pass, grope as you make your way around. On the next, just tease with your fingernails. Draw circles around your areola and nipples. Pinch and tug at them, or have your partner kiss, lick, or suck them.

Tease your inner thighs, but don't touch your vulva. Much like when you were exploring your erogenous zones, get as close to your vulva as you can, and then pull back. Use every erogenous zone you know you have to your advantage. If you're exploring with your partner, have them kiss your neck or touch your breasts while teasing your thighs and hips. Use those zones to your advantage. Keep doing that, each time getting a little bit closer to touching yourself, but pull back each time until you feel like you might explode if you don't touch yourself.

5. Use enhancements. On many sex toy websites, there will be a recommended product known as 'clit sensitizer,' 'enhancer gel,' or 'arousal gel.' They are designed to increase your clit's sensitivity and make it easier to achieve orgasm or make your orgasms that much more intense. This can help if you feel like you need a lot of stimulation to get close to that climax or have trouble climaxing with your partner. Use carefully and as

directed. Most recommend you apply a small dab to your clit 10-15 minutes before sex. It'll feel a little cold and a bit tingly at first. But once you start to have sex, you'll feel the difference.

6. Take advantage of the G-Spot. The infamous g-spot, or Gräfenberg spot named after the German gynecologist who found it, can often aid in reaching orgasm. Some women do report that they have reached orgasm through g-spot stimulation alone. But if you're still in the process of exploring your body, both the g-spot and clit should be used in tandem. This spot is located approximately 2 to 3 inches, about your index finger's length, along the upward-facing wall of the vagina. Putting added pressure on this part of the vagina can be immensely pleasurable during sex or masturbation.

The g-spot is also known as the Skene's Gland or urethral sponge. It's the slightly spongier part of the vagina that rests up against the wall between the vagina and the urethra. This gland is what's responsible for female ejaculation or squirting. It's also known as the female prostate.

A note on squirting: if you find you are a woman who can squirt, you do not need to worry about peeing on your partner. The liquid isn't urine. The liquid that your body expels during squirting is anatomically the same fluid that's in male ejaculate. That's why the Skene's Gland is called the female prostate.

Manipulating the g-sport during masturbation or foreplay can be extremely pleasurable. If you stimulate your clit simultaneously, it could be that much easier to reach orgasm with your partner. If you're going to attempt to squirt, put down a towel or use sheets you don't care for. This is some messy work. Have them use their fingers inside of you, curling up against the spongey upper wall, and thrust while you use your fingers or a toy against your clit. Work together at a rhythm that feels best to you and pay attention to how you're feeling. If you start to get the feeling like you have to pee, that's completely natural as your partner is putting pressure on your urethra through the g-spot. If you're not in any pain, don't stop.

If you're both working at the same rhythm, you should feel a pressure building until your partner can't keep their fingers inside of you anymore. When they pull out, some clear liquid might come out. Congratulations. You can squirt.

Female ejaculation is not an orgasm, however. The two are not as closely tied as they are with men. Even after you've squirted, keep stimulating your clit. You should be even more sensitive than before it, and it will be even easier to get to that peak.

If you can't get yourself to the point of ejaculation, that's okay. If you found the experience pleasurable, there's no harm in continuing to try. Not every woman can, and not every woman can squirt the same amount. Some don't even realize that they did until they get up, and there's a big puddle where their butt was sitting. Other women can have some geyser-like experience. The Skene's Gland can hold anywhere from a few droplets of liquid to almost a quarter of a cup.

Not everyone is going to get to squirt on their first try. If it's something on your Want list, keep experimenting. Try differing positions, different speeds, or other toys. Your partner's fingers might not be enough, and you find that you need more internal stimulation. See if you can find a g-spot vibrator that you like to get you right where you need it. Use a vibrator on your clit instead of your fingers. A lot of women have found success with squirting will using air pulsation stimulators. Having that extra suction on their clit helps women get closer to that point of squirting.

Having an Orgasm During Sex
If you listened to the advice in Chapter 2, then you'll already know that sex means more than penetration. It can be anything that you deem intimate with your significant other. But if you are having trouble reaching orgasm during penetration with your partner, and that's something you'd like to fix, there are some strategies you can try and see what works best for you.

Much like when you masturbate, the focus of sex does not have to be on having an orgasm. It's nice to have, and it certainly makes you feel happier and closer to your partner when you reach it. But if it's all you're thinking about. If your mind is so focused on getting to that orgasm to show your partner you're having a good time, you're missing the point, and that orgasm is going to get further and further away from you.

Focus on the moment. Focus on how your partner is making you feel. Are they touching you in a way that feels good? Are they whispering something in your ear to get you turned on? If you're too focused on your orgasm to notice how wonderful the moment is right now, your priorities are in the wrong place.

That being said, with the right communication, techniques, and tools, you can achieve orgasm during sex. Being open to the possibility that it won't happen works like reversal psychology on your body. You've accepted that you might not get an orgasm, so your body is open to more touches and sensations that get you to that goal that much easier.

Before you being penetrative sex, how much time did you spend on foreplay? Do you feel sufficiently turned on? On average, it takes women up to 4 times as long as men to reach orgasm. You might just need more time to get turned on and warmed up.

Start ahead of the game with orgasms. Talk with your partner about having them make you orgasm as part of foreplay. Decide how you want to do that, with a toy, your partner's fingers, oral sex, etc. Once you've reached an orgasm, your body is extra sensitive, and it's that much easier to reach an orgasm with your partner. Set yourself up for success and get a head start on your partner. If you discover that you're multi-orgasmic, it could be a part of the fun, seeing how many times your partner can make you orgasm before you even come close to penetrative sex.

Are you getting enough clitoral stimulation? As mentioned above, most women cannot reach orgasm through penetration alone. The inner branches of the clit make it feel terrific, but they're not likely to get you to orgasm all on their own. Have your partner play with your clit a little bit during sex or play with it yourself. Your partner will most likely be turned on watching you please yourself, making the sex that much better for both of you.

Try a different position. Some positions will lend themselves to more clitoral stimulation than others. If you are on top, your clit is going to grid against your partner's stomach and hips as you move. If you're trying out doggy style, if you're flat on the bed, your pelvis will be able to grind against the bed, or you can get your hand between your legs more freely and play with your clit in time with your partner's thrusts.

It's all about timing. If you're going too fast on your clit and your partner is thrusting slow and deep, it might feel good, but it might also feel off. Sync your rhythms together, make your whole vulva work in tandem to get you to immense pleasure. Ask your partner to slow down or speed up. Slow your own fingers down or turn the setting on your toy down so that it isn't too intense. It is possible to overstimulate yourself, and that doesn't feel good. You can always build up if something doesn't feel like it's enough. Once you've overstimulated yourself, you have to pull way back and build up all over again. It's better to take your time, find the rhythm that works best for both of you, and have fun.

See? The female orgasm isn't as mysterious as it used to be. You just need to take the time to learn your body and figure out what you like. Women are taught early on that they shouldn't explore and touch themselves. It's not ladylike. But all that does is breed a generation of adult women who don't even know they can achieve such pleasure.

Take these tools, tips, techniques, and suggestions, and find what works for you. Find what you like and what you don't. Share these new discoveries with your partner and see what they would be willing to explore with you. Once you've opened the floodgates of sexual exploration, there's no closing them. There's always something new to learn, try, or play with.

Even after discovering what you like, there will always be some new position you never thought of trying that is better than the last. You never stop learning.

CHAPTER 5: GAMES TO PLAY DURING FOREPLAY

Games to Play With Your Clothes On:
The No Hands Game.

Sit beside your partner and start kissing. The kisses can be sweet and sensual, deep and slow, or teasing pecks all over their body. The game has one rule: You cannot use your hands. Every other part of your body is fair game. You could use your whole body to grind against your partner, your mouth to take their clothes off, or just kiss the hell out of them until they've had enough. The possibilities are endless when the rules of the game are simple.

Whoever puts their hands on the other first is the loser and therefore gets punished. It's up to you how you want to dole out punishments. Maybe the first person to give in has to do the dishes for the whole week or vacuum the entire house. You couple play the game in rounds like a stripping game. The first person to give in and use their hands has to remove an article of clothing. One round at a time until one or both of you is naked.

Find the "inserts food item here."

For this game, you'll need two things: a blindfold and a sticky substance of your choice. You can play this game with your clothes on or clothes off. Have your partner put something over their eyes and take your food, for explanation's sake, let's say chocolate syrup, and dab a little bit of it somewhere on your body. It can be somewhere accessible for them to find, like on your neck or breasts. Or it can be somewhere a bit harder for them to find, like between your fingers or behind your ear.

Your partner's goal is to find this dab of chocolate through any means necessary within the parameters you've set. You can make it a rule that you can only use your lips, no hands. Or set a timer and see if your partner can find the chocolate within the time set. Play it like a game of HORSE. Whenever you fail to find the chocolate, you get a letter or a point. Trade-off who has to find the chocolate within the timer set. Whoever fails to find it five or more times loses and suffers the consequences.

If you want to make this even harder, play while you still have some clothes on, preferably clothes you don't care about getting dirty. Then your partner has to determine if it's worth it to check under your clothing for the chocolate and waste time or continue to search elsewhere and risk missing the treasure entirely. Make it a sexy scavenger hunt, and your body is the map.

Strip Poker/Card Game:

This is one of the most iconic foreplay games. There are many variations, but the most common is to play a round of poker, then the loser has to remove an article of clothing. The game continues until someone is naked, and the winner gets to enjoy their spoils.

If you want the game to last longer, you could add an incentive to win, rather than just punishment for losing. For every losing hand, you must remove one article of clothing. Additionally, with every winning hand, you get to put one piece of clothing back on.

It makes the game last much longer that way, and it draws out the anticipation of getting to the end.

Someone could be losing for the entire game, be nearly down to their panties, but then with a stroke of luck, they start to win every hand. Clothing comes back on, and their partner ends up being the loser. With these rules, there's no telling how long the game could last.

To add even more stakes to your game, add wagers. Instead of merely making the loser remove an article of clothing, wager what you'll remove, or what the loser will have to do for you when they lose. Start with wagering a piece of clothing; then, you can raise and add more clothing to the mix. Such as suggesting, "I wager my pants," then your partner could go, "I see pants and raise you a sock." And so on. If all you wager is clothing, you could be naked after one hand if you keep raising the stakes. If you want this game to go longer, set a cap on how much you can wager per round. Only allow each of you to raise a maximum of 2 times so the game keeps going.

Add more items to the pot like sexual favors. "I wager my shirt and a hand job," "I see your offer and raise you a blow job." Then if you lose, you take off your shirt, and you owe your partner those favors at their determined time. It could be right then and there, or whenever they desire.

You can take the principle of 'lose a round and strip' and apply it to any game you and your partner like. Maybe you two are more Mario Kart or racing game fans. Whoever comes in last has to take off an article of clothing. If you want to add an extra incentive to win, make it so whoever wins gets to pick which article of clothing it is.

Question Games

Truth or Dare isn't just for girls at a slumber party. You and your partner can enjoy a sexy version of this. Give Truth or Kiss or Truth or Strip a try. Or turn it up a notch with Truth, Dare, or Strip. Write down some questions ahead of time, or do a web search for 'sexy truth or dare questions.' Take turns asking each other 'truth or dare?' If your partner chooses Truth, ask them a question on the list. If they do not wish to answer, they immediately have to take off one article of clothing of your choosing. The same goes for the Dare option. If they don't complete the dare, they lose another piece of clothing.

The Dares can be as small as 'prank call your mom,' or they can be much sexier. Maybe dare your partner to grind against the couch while you videotape it. If your partner consents, you're good to go. If they don't want to follow through with the dare, they're down one article of clothing.

Games to Create Endless Possibilities

Sex dice are a common way to get acquainted with your partner's body. One die has body parts, usually erogenous zones, on each side. The other die has actions such as kiss, suck, slap, or grope. You or your partner rolls the dice and does whatever comes up if it's feasible. If you roll and the dice tell you to lick your partner's nipple, that's what you do. Occasionally you may end up with something less than desirable like 'spank neck.' In those cases, just laugh it off and roll again. It's all about having fun in the bedroom with your partner.

Playing with Sex dice is a great way to get to know your partner's erogenous zones. If you don't want to worry about the action die, just roll the die with body parts and do whatever you want with whichever body part it lands. If you land on 'neck' kiss and suck on your partner's neck, maybe give them a hickey if they're okay with that. If you roll it and it comes up, 'butt,' try some light spanks or groping. Try anything you can think of and see if it feels good.

Fatebowl

Get two bowls or cups and tear up some paper into 20 foldable strips. Each of you should write down ten things you want to do your partner or want them to do to you. Grab a set of dice, and each of you takes a turn throwing it. Whoever rolls the lowest number has to choose from their 'bowl of fate' filled with items from their partner and see what they will now have to endure. What you put on the paper doesn't have to be sexual. You could have written 'massage,' 'vacuum the house in a thong,' 'get ten spanks,' or 'wash the toilet.' It can be anything that comes to mind. The fun in this game is in the chance to retaliate. The more ridiculous the tasks, the more fun it is when the loser gets their chance to get back at their partner.

You can make the game entirely sexual, or just playful. It's up to you and what kind of game you want to foster. Playing in the bedroom should be fun. It doesn't have to all be grunting and grinding. Making your partner eat you out while they're wearing a pirate's eyepatch is all part of the fun and games that can make sex great. You have to be able to laugh at yourself and with your partner. Intentionally make these games as ridiculous as possible, so when something awkward comes up, it doesn't seem like that big of a deal. You already got the most embarrassing thing out of the way early on in the evening.

Games to Help You Get Ideas

Read erotica together. You can find a variety of it on the internet. Search for any possible erotic scenario, and you'll find a website or two populated with these kinds of stories. Literotica is a good source of free erotic fiction. They can be well written and literary, or over the top and ridiculous. It doesn't matter as long as they're sexy.

Either come prepared with your own story to read aloud to your partner or take turns reading from the same text. Split up the characters, so it's like you're taking on the story together and breathing a new life into through your interpretation. If the story is less than spectacularly written, give the characters funny voices to make it more interesting. Nothing is more intimate than being able to laugh with one another.

Rule 34 of the internet: if it exists, there's porn for it. If there's a particular movie or tv franchise, you and your partner like search on websites like fanfiction.net or Archive of Our Own for your show or movie and the characters you'd want. You can filter by rating, if you're looking for erotica, filter for Explicit content, and even add some actions into the tags to find just the right story for you.

You could read a story about Doctor Who having a romp with one of his companions on a planet and in a time far far away.

Or read about how Iron Man and Pepper Potts conceived their daughter. If there's an idea you've had about any fictional character, there is a good chance that the same story exists on the internet. Good or bad? You decide.

Red light, Greenlight

This is an excellent game to play when you're getting to know each other's erogenous zones. There are apps and websites you can find that will set a timer, and each time it's set, the time goes up a little bit. Set the timer, and take turns touching each other for as long as the timer is going. You can be teasing their neck, or their hips, or giving them a hand job.

Most importantly, when the timer goes off, you stop. It doesn't matter how good it feels or how much you both want to continue. You pull away and don't let your partner pull you back in. Then you set the timer again, and now it's your partner's turn. The game ends when one of you has an orgasm, or you just can't take it anymore, and you two start going at it.

If you want to make the game even more interesting, do a round of rock, paper, and scissors to determine who will be the one to be touched for the timer's duration. That way, no one gets a fair amount of time to cool down. You could be bad at rock, paper, scissors, and lose every time, so your partner toys with you for every round until you orgasm.

If you choose to go the route of 'first to orgasm loses' determine what the punishment will be. Does the winner get to do whatever they want with the loser? Or does the loser have to do something for the winner? That's entirely up to you. Confer to your Want and Will lists and see what you can come up with to raise the stakes and see how long you can stave off orgasm.

Temperature play:

You most likely saw beginner bondage and BDSM kits when the two of you were looking for toys. Amongst those were likely candles meant for play with hot wax or molds for ice cubes. Be very careful when adding temperature play to your foreplay. Start with cold, and then work your way up to hot.

Take an ice cube and rub it over your partner's nipples, down their side, up their thigh, anywhere you think they might be sensitive. Pay special attention to how they move, what they say, and if they enjoy it. Ice play isn't for everyone; some people feel nothing; some people don't like it at all.

If you're going to go the way of hot wax, do so carefully and slowly. Use candles designed for this kind of play. Light the candle and carefully drip the wax over your partner's body. The wax is hot at first, but as it cools, the area gets hypersensitive. Don't focus on one spot for too long, and talk to your partner.
If something is too painful, stop, and reassess what you can change.

No matter how you choose to play, the possibilities are endless. Use these games to learn each other's bodies and extend the intimacy. Sex is playful, and that should extend through to your foreplay. Have fun with it and explore the possibilit

CHAPTER 6: ORAL SEX

Oral sex, by definition, is sex. Much like foreplay does not have to be treated as the opening act, oral sex be is the main event. It can be sensual, sweet, and loving. It can be rough, lustful, and passionate. By engaging in oral sex, you're participating in something just as intimate as penetrative sex. You are more open, more vulnerable, and more intense you could ever imagine.

Oral Sex on a Woman

For many women, oral sex is an excellent way for them to begin orgasming with a partner. Additionally, for many women, this is why they haven't achieved that yet. Women are taught from a young age to be ashamed of what lies between their legs and never show it to another. They are taught that their pleasure is derived from their partner's pleasure. Or worse, they're taught that their pleasure doesn't exist at all.

Orgasm through oral sex is fantastic. The sensations brought about through it are unparalleled in any other sexual experience. Oral doesn't just involve the mouth. It can include hands, fingers, tongues, lips, and anything else your partner can think of that also involves using their mouth.

Using oral sex as a precursor to penetration is a great way to get your body primed to have an orgasm with your partner. If you're a multi-orgasmic woman or can have multiple orgasms in a row, you and your partner can go right from oral to penetration without much time in between. Once you've had an orgasm, it's that much easier to reach that peak again.

Oral sex, like other forms of sex, is all in the technique. And it differs from person to person. Like it was mentioned earlier, every woman responds to sexual stimulus differently. Take the time to work with your partner and learn what makes you both happy, pleased, and comfortable.

The position makes a big difference. Try as many as you can think of. Lay on your back with your partner between your legs. Lie on your stomach with your hips raised and your partner behind you. Try straddling your partner's face if you feel like you have a supportive enough headboard and sufficient core strength. Sit on the edge of the bed with your partner between your legs, kneeling on the floor. Use pillows to lift your hips so your partner can try for another angle or to ease any pressure on your partner's knees.

Test out what feels best for you. You can either try multiple positions in one night or make it a game. Try a different position every night until you find the one position that feels right to you, and that brings you the most pleasure and comfort.

When performing oral sex on a woman, don't just focus on one area of the vulva. The clit feels good, but not if that's your primary focus. The entire genital region is one large erogenous zone. Work all of the angles. Tease the labia. Slip your tongue slightly inside of her, then pull back. Start by touching everywhere but the clit until you can't stop yourself.

Tease the clit lightly. Give it a swipe of the tongue, then pull back and focus on other areas. Make your partner as sensitive as possible when you do finally reach her clit.

Don't just go for one pattern and repeat it non-stop. Try different designs with your tongue with every swipe. First, try moving your tongue in circles. Then in a triangle. After that, try spelling out the alphabet with your tongue. Pay attention to how she moves when you do a particular shape with your tongue. After you change up the tactics, pull back, leave her wanting more, then go back in and repeat a rhythm that she liked. Alternate with the new and the familiar.

Use your lips as well as your tongue. If suction is something your partner likes, try lightly sucking on her clit between licks. Suck harder or suck softer. Use your lips on her labia surrounding her vaginal opening. The whole area is sensitive, after all. Take advantage of it.

Use your fingers. Oral sex on a woman isn't just the use of the mouth. Use your hands. Pull her thighs apart. Lift them up onto your shoulders so that you can get closer. Finger her while you suck on or lick at her clit. Some women like to feel external and internal stimulation at the same time. Curl your fingers up to tease her g-spot as you time your thrusts with the flick of your tongue. Move between rhythms. Go softer, then harder, then fainter again.

It's good to experiment with fingers and how many your partner can take. Not every woman likes the stretching feeling of having too many fingers inside of her. Start with one and work your way up. The average woman enjoys the feeling of two fingers.

Take your cues from your partner. Ask them what feels good and what doesn't feel right. Ask them if there's anything they want to change. She might want more tongue or more fingers inside of her. She might want you to play with her breasts while you're pleasuring her. Women get aroused with their whole bodies. Turn your partner's entire body into one big erogenous zone.

If you're fingering her while eating her out, you'll likely start to feel a tightness on your fingers when she is close to orgasm. Keep going. Just because she's clenching, it doesn't mean she's orgasming yet. It just means she's close. When she gets there, you'll know. Keep doing what you're doing and get ready. If you're close to her vulva, watch for her hips. Make sure they don't hit you in the face. If you feel so inclined, pin her hips down as you finger her and watch as she unravels before you.

When she's done with her orgasm, ask her what she needs, what she wants. Some women are ready to go for penetration right after an orgasm; some aren't. Your partner might need a break before continuing further play. Get her some water, then get ready for more fun.

If her pleasure isn't enough to get you going, there's no harm in touching yourself while you're eating her out. She'll be turned on because you're turned on. You'll be even more turned on because she is turned on; it's a win-win. If you two are feeling adventurous, you might want to give the 69 position a try.

This position is where you both perform oral sex on each other at the same time. The name creates a particular mental image, but it doesn't necessarily have to mean that one of you is right on top of the other. You can easily, and sometimes more comfortably, enjoy this position lying on your sides. This way, you can both rest your neck on your partner's thigh or the pillow and increase your pleasure that much more before you won't be worrying about neck pains. If you want to try being one on top of the other, maximum safety, let the partner who is performing oral sex on the partner with the penis be on top. It allows them easy access to move their head freely if they find they have difficulty breathing or swallowing. Feeling trapped isn't sexy unless you like that.

Oral Sex on a Man
Performing oral sex on men is slightly more straight forward for men than it is for women. But that doesn't mean you should get stuck in a rut and going through the motions to get your partner off. With a little creativity, you can find plenty of new ways to please your partner without just sticking his penis in your mouth.

It's important to remember that the whole penis is sensitive. Make sure it gets as much love and attention as possible. Use your hand where necessary, but let your mouth guide the action. Your hand is merely following. As discussed earlier, the penis and the clit were the same organs in development. As the head of the clit is extremely sensitive, so is the head of the penis. It's vital not to overstimulate it, but it should get its own tender loving care.

Get into a rhythm and find what your partner likes. Once it feels like they've gotten used to that rhythm, switch things up. Slow down, speed up, just use your tongue along the shaft. Do anything to change up the rhythm to keep your partner guessing.

With your partner's permission, bring his scrotum into play. If it's something you want or are willing to do, play with them in your hand as you run your mouth up and down the shaft of his penis. You might even want to try licking and sucking on them while you use your hand to stroke him. Pay attention to his cues and ask him if he likes something. While the motions are straight forward, not every man likes every rhythm and sensation. Communication is key.

When your partner is about to orgasm, it's especially important to have somewhere for the semen to go. This should be something you've talked about beforehand. Do you want to swallow it? Would you rather he finish on your chest or in your hand? For many men, having their partner swallow can increase the pleasure for them. And for many women, swallowing can add a sense of empowerment to their play. It's all up to the both of you. Do that which you want or are willing, and play safely.

General Oral Sex Tips
No matter who's genitals are involved, the best tip for good oral sex is: practice good personal hygiene. This doesn't just mean waxing. It means keeping your mouth free from disease as well. There are many mucus membranes involved in oral sex, and everyone involved must be clean and healthy.

Ladies, you do not need to have a waxed clean vulva so that your partner will engage in oral sex. Pubic hair is essential for the overall cleanliness of your genitals. But if you don't want to have a full bush, you can trim your hair with a bikini trimmer. The vagina is like a self-cleaning oven. It has a delicate balance and has a natural way of getting rid of excess bacteria. You do not need to cleanse it. Your vulva should taste like a vulva. Leave the cleansers and the douches at the store. You don't need them. There have been women who claim that they can make their vulvas taste sweeter by eating excessive amounts of pineapple, but it's not recommended you try this. Your vulva is pleasing as it is.

Men, trim your pubic hair. If you want to foster an experience that is fun for both of you, this is the most straightforward step. Pubic hair is essential for your overall health, but there's nothing wrong with trimming it down so that it doesn't get in the way of your pleasure. And clean your penis. If you've had an active day, take a shower before you being your bedroom playtime. Your partner will thank you.

It's okay to have hang-ups about your body and feel self-conscious about having your partner's face so close to your genitals. It's a section of your body that someone taught you from a young age that you should keep secret and private. It's easy not to worry about it when you're both under the sheets, and you don't have to think much about it. But when your partner is coming face to face with the most intimate part of your body, it's easy to get self-conscious. Just relax and trust that your partner is performing oral sex on you because they want to. There's no need to worry. Lie back, take a few deep breaths, and enjoy.

If anything is still troubling you about having your partner down between your legs, talk to them and figure out where your hang-ups are. Work with them so you know how to fix them and can further enjoy your time together.

Ways to Make your Oral Sex More Exciting

If you've gotten the basics down and want a little more, there are always games you can play and things you can add to make it that much more exciting.

Use edible paints. Often on sex toy retailer websites, there are toys for oral sex. One of them is edible paints. These are usually kits that come with multi-colored chocolate and a brush that you can use to paint works of art on your partner and then lick them clean. Check the ingredients and materials to ensure there is nothing you or your partner are allergic to and have fun. Put the paints all over your partner's body and enjoy the sensation of running your tongue along their body. Be careful not to put too much directly on the vulva or penis if you plan to have sex afterward. Excess sugar isn't good for the vagina's natural ph balance. It's just good clean, messy, fun.

Try doing something while your partner is performing oral sex on you. Try reading a book, singing a song, anything that requires a bit of focus while your partner is performing oral sex on you. See how long you can go without breaking your concentration. Your partner will have fun, making it harder for you to keep your focus while trying that much harder to keep it. See how long you can go without orgasming. Make that final peak of pleasure your breaking point, if you can.

Try edging. Edging is the practice of getting you or your partner to that very peak of orgasm, and then pulling back. Over and over again. Oral sex is a fantastic avenue to start trying edging. Once you and your partner have found each other's rhythms, you'll have plenty of fun getting each other right to the peak of orgasm before you pull back and watch them squirm. Then you can watch them as you push them back up to that brink over and over again until you finally let them have that release that they want.

Oral sex is dependent on communication. Talk to each other before, during, and throughout. Experiment with that feels right to you and what seems good on paper to spice things up. Something you'd been doing all along might be a real turn off for your partner. You must voice these concerns to improve and keep your sex life happy and exciting. More importantly, tell them what felt good. Communication should always be about encouraging your partner and telling them when something needs to be adjusted. You just have to find that balance that works for your partnership and your bedroom.

CHAPTER 7: ROLE-PLAY

Roleplaying is an excellent way to bring more whimsy and fun into your bedroom time. Sex should be fun. You should be able to play together. And in some cases, that can mean that you're playing entirely different people. Roleplaying can take many forms, but the most common is character role-play. There is also scenario-based role-play and control based role-play. All of these kinds of play are unique and have their own set of rules and guidelines so that you and your partner stay safe.

When entering into a role-play headspace, it's essential to talk things through with your partner beforehand. Talk about what you want to happen and what you don't want to happen. Make sure you're on the same page with each other, and you've worked out your safe word or another exit strategy before you begin playing.

Go over your Want, Will, and Won't lists and see if any of the games or acts you want to try would work well with the certain role-play you have in mind. If you're role-playing as characters from a show or movie you like, how would those characters act? Would they be into bondage? You're putting on a play for the two of you. You are the cast, directors, and audience all in one. Make sure you think through all of the possibilities before you begin. All decisions have to be unanimous.

It's okay to put some things into the 'will' category. Maybe you say that 'if it feels right at the moment for you to spank me, I'm okay with that. But unless I ask you to, I don't want it.' It's okay to set that boundary before you start the game.

Before you begin any role-play scenario, it's important to go over with your partner what you are okay with and what you are not okay with happening. Getting into a role-play headspace can be incredibly intimate, and it can also be extremely vulnerable. You need to have your safe words decided on before you get anywhere near the bedroom.

Character-Based Role-play

As the name would suggest, these role-play scenarios are rooted in the characters you and your partner create or the ones you borrow from other franchises. These can be your stereotypical 'repairman and housewife who doesn't have any money to pay you,' or the 'fireman who saved you from a burning building and there's only one way to thank him' sorts of scenarios.

You can even draw from characters you already know. Maybe you and your partner are very into Sherlock Holmes, and you want to play around as Sherlock and Watson, reenact a scene from the show, and give it the ending you want. Or act out any fan fiction you might have read together. These sorts of role-plays have endless possibilities. You just have to open your minds.

Character-based role-play can start well before the bedroom. You and your partner could go out to a club or a restaurant and pretend to be completely different people. Act as though you are strangers meeting for the very first time. Pretend that it's your first date all over again and recapture that spark you felt when you first met. Do your best to stay in character the whole time. Have a name, occupation, and backstory ready for your character so you can stay in the headspace for as long as possible. It's okay to break character if you have to. It's a game. It's meant to be fun.

If you're going to go the 'pick each other up in a bar' route, decide where you want to play. This could be a chance to try a whole new location. Meet up in a hotel bar and book a room for you to play in. Pretend you're two people from out of town who meet up and end up having a one night stand. If you're going to meet up at a bar and drink a little, get a cab or rideshare for your rides there and back so you can both be safe and maybe fool around a little and make out in the back seat on your way back to your home.

If you want to make it feel as though you could be caught any second, pretend that your husband or wife will be home any second, and you have to get these urges out soon. With this kind of play, it's important to discuss how it makes you feel afterward.

See if you can both stay in character throughout the sex. Maybe even set a punishment for the first person to break character. Play question games in character like 'Truth, Dare, or Strip." Get into the character and how they would react to the situation. Would your character be outgoing? Would they be timid? Is this your character's first time with a new partner since a messy break-up? Is this their first time with another person entirely? These are important to think about when you're coming up with a character for your role-play.

Under character role-play, there is a subset best described as 'scenario-based role-play.' This kind of role-play combines elements of character play but with a twist. Usually, this will involve you and your partner as yourselves but in a different scenario. You can add a power dynamic to your play like 'boss and secretary,' or 'teacher-student.' This is much more focused on the scenario and the power dynamic involved in that rather than your characters themselves.

This kind of role-play also lends into a bit of control play. Most likely, the scenario you're going to come up with will be one in which one of you is in a position of power over the other. Work out how you want that dynamic to play into the scenario, what names you're okay being called, and what you want your partner to do, with, or for you. A good scenario is best in the details.

With any of these role-plays, have fun with clothing and costume pieces. Do up your hair in a new way that better fits your character and try new sexy clothes. If you're going for a student and teacher role-play, try putting your hair in pigtails. If you're the teacher, put on one of your best suits, or at least an outfit that you don't mind getting wrinkled.

If you're going for a boss and secretary role-play, get out a button-up shirt that makes you feel good and play it up to be sexier. It's okay for it to feel a little pornographic. You're acting out your own porn with your partner, and you two are the audience. Make it fun for you.

If it's helpful to get ideas, watch porn together, or read erotica together. Not only will it help you both get turned on, but it'll also give you ideas for your own role-plays. It's okay to laugh at the outlandish things that the actors are doing on screen and want to reenact them in some way that's comfortable for you.

Be the boss showing the secretary how to type up correctly and send an email. Show your troublesome student what happens to students who don't get good grades. Be the personal trainer who is just trying to help your client have good form when performing a squat. In some cases, the more ridiculous, the better. Be playful, be honest, and have fun.

Control Based Role-play
Control based role-play requires the most amount of communication before, during, and after playtime. As the name would suggest, this kind of roleplay involves one person to give up control and the other to take overpower. Anything you do in this scenario should come from your Want or Will list. These kinds of role-play scenarios can be very intense, and they're not for everyone. It's okay to decide that it's not for you after you've given it a try with your partner. Communicate, see how you can make it better for you, and what you can take out so that you are both that much happier.

Control based role-play bases itself in the BDSM culture. BDSM stands for Bondage and Discipline, Domination and Submission, and Sadism and Masochism. It encompasses a wide variety of kinks and toys. For the purposes of a control-based role play, the focus will be on the Dominance and Submission aspect of the acronym.

In a dominant and submissive roleplay, one partner will take on the dominant role while the other takes on the part of the submissive. The dominant sets the rules and enforces the laws, the submissive follows. You can set up this scenario however you want. Think about switching up the roles every once in a while,

73

if you wish, to switch things up and see how it feels from the other side.

Traditionally, people who are more inclined to be control freaks or need to organize every detail of their day prefer to be submissive. They find it incredibly freeing to give up control in such a primal sense. But, despite how it may look at first glance, the submissive has all of the power in the dynamic. Sure, they may be the ones following orders and getting punished if they don't follow them correctly. But nothing happens without the submissive's consent. Nothing happens that they have not agreed to before beginning the scene, and the submissive can end the scene at any time by saying 'red' or his or her safe word.

It's the job of the dominant to pay attention to their submissive and take note of when they may not be enjoying something as much as they should. It's okay to stop and reassess as long as you both feel safe and cared for. The dominant has the control. They guide the scene and their submissive, but they still answer to their submissive.

Aspects of this sort of play can include the other letters of the acronym, especially bondage. It's a popular tool when it comes to domination. If you purchased a beginner BDSM toy kit, you'd have plenty to help you get started. Your kit likely came with rope or handcuffs, start there and see what you like.

Figure out what aspects of the domination or submission appeal most to you. Like with character role-play, you might have a new name. Many dominants like their submissives to call them Master or Mistress, while some like to keep things simple with

Sir or Ma'am. Work out with your partner what works best for you.

This sort of role-playing can be very freeing for couples. It allows them to tap into more primal instincts and urges that they would not have otherwise voiced. It's easy to get lost in these kinds of scenes. That is why it's so important to have an exit strategy. You can easily get lost in the pleasure and forget your boundaries until they cross them. If things go too far, say your safe word loudly and clearly, and discuss what you can fix.

If you want to dig a little deeper into the dominant and submissive headspace, there subset known as DdLg, or Daddy Dom, Little Girl, is something worth researching. This extends beyond the bedroom for some people, but it doesn't have to if that's not something you're comfortable doing. It can be as simple as calling your partner 'daddy' in bed and leave it at that. This subset of domination creates a very vulnerable space that not every person or couple is comfortable with or ready for. If it intrigues you, put it on your Will or Want list. If this does not appeal to you at all, put it on your Won't list so you and your partner know where you stand. Every aspect of control based role-play needs discussing ahead of time, and this one is crucial.

For control based role-play to be successful, everything needs negotiating ahead of time. It may seem unsexy to talk out every possibility before you get down and dirty. Still, it's better to talk it through before you start than leave some gray areas unspoken and discover a new rigid boundary in the middle of playtime. If that should happen, you need to feel safe enough to stop the action and figure out what is not working. But the likelihood of that happening is lessened if you've talked through all possible scenarios ahead of time.

Start slowly. Maybe at first, you'll start by only using the role-play personas during foreplay, and then when you move on to more sex, you drop them and let your regular dynamic take place. Gradually add it to more and more of your playtime until you're in a place where you're comfortable holding onto the dynamic until you're completely done for the night. No matter how long you keep the scene for, you need to discuss it afterward.

There will be a whole chapter on aftercare at the end of the book, but it's of the utmost importance when you engage in control-based role-play. It strengthens your connection to your partner and lets the submissive feel comfortable and safe. When dealing with these kinds of role-plays, aftercare is non-negotiable. It is a mandatory step.

It's common for people filling the submissive role to feel very vulnerable during and after a scene. For some, they may not want to be touched afterward. They may wish to cuddle afterward. Once you've finished for the night, a simple 'what do you need' is all you need to ask of your partner. Get them a glass of water, a fuzzy blanket, or their favorite pillow. Do whatever you need to do to make them comfortable, safe, and loved.

If you used new words or called each other by new names during your scene, talk about how they made you feel. Some people like being called a slut or a whore during intense role-play scenes but don't you dare call them that outside of the bedroom. Talk to each other and see how the scene felt to you during and afterward. You may have liked something during the scene, but you don't want to do it again in hindsight. Maybe the spanks felt good, but now that you've finished, your butt hurts, and next time you want your partner to spank you lighter. Talk it out and negotiate so that you both can feel the most pleasure you can.

Role-play is a great way to take the familiar and tweak it just enough to make it brand new and extraordinary. Pretending to be another person can bring out a whole new side of you that you never knew existed. It gives you the freedom to try out new kinks and ways to play with your partner. It gives you the freedom to be playful, silly, and a little pornographic. The only limits are the edges of your imagination. Pick a character, location, scene, or punishment. Go from there.

CHAPTER 8: MORE GAMES

Every time you introduce something new into the bedroom, it should be a unanimous decision. You and your partner need to agree that it is something you want to bring into the bedroom for this first time. After you've tried it that first time, you can assess if you liked it if you didn't like it, and if there's any way you can change it to make it that much more pleasurable should you try again.

Go over your safe words and make sure both of you are on the same page. If you're going to be trying something that may impede your ability to speak, such as trying a gag, come up with a secondary, non-verbal way to tell each other that you need to slow down. If your hands are tied, and you have a gag in your mouth, maybe if you bang your foot on the bed three times, that means you need to stop. Work that out before you get started on anything, so you both know what is and isn't okay.

Good playtime relies on everything that happens to be safe and consensual. When you trust your partner to keep you safe and know that they will not be hurt if you want to stop something, you open your mind and your body to so much more pleasure.

Bondage Play
If you've been interested in bondage and don't know where to start, the best place to start is the beginning. Start as slowly as you can and build up from there. Start with just binding your hands together, then move them in different positions. Figure out if you prefer to have your hands tied in front of you, behind you, or over your head. Do you like having them bound while

you're on your back or your front? When you're comfortable with that, try binding them to the bed if you can. See how that feels. Each time, be checking in with your partner to see how each other is feeling and if something needs to change. Maybe the rope is chafing you, and you'd rather use a softer fabric.

You don't even need a fancy bondage kit or handcuffs to try bondage. Take any piece of fabric: a necktie, a scarf, the sleeve of your shirt, and get started experimenting. When you've determined that you like bondage at all, then you can spend money on a beginning BDSM kit or friendlier methods of bondage. Walk before you run

When you've gotten comfortable with binding your hands, decide if you want to move onto securing your legs. What would you need to do that? Is that something you like? Bondage, when focused on the legs, usually involves keeping them spread apart. Decide for yourself if that kind of vulnerability is something you can do. If not, that's okay. You can like bondage and just like your hands tied up. That's entirely up to you. You're playing a game, and it should be fun. If it's not fun or doesn't add to your pleasure, it's on the Won't list.

More advanced forms of bondage, known as shibari, bind the rope or fabric in very intricate knots over your partner's body. The fun comes not only from tying them up but in releasing them. The one tied up can feel an immense amount of pleasure from having the rope slide across their skin or feeling their partner's hands against them as they are bound. Make sure to do your research before trying any kind of intricate knotting. You need to know how to tie the knots correctly for maximum safety.

The teasing in getting your partner tied up is a lot of fun, but you should be able to untie your partner quickly if something goes wrong and your partner needs to be released.

Bondage relies on an immense amount of trust. You are giving up complete control of the movement of your body to your partner. It's essential to establish that trust before you play, determine how tightly your partner will bind you, and what you need to say to get them to untie you. When you're finished, discuss with your partner what you liked and what you didn't. And determine what you want to try again.

As mentioned above, sensory deprivation is a big part of bondage. Most commonly, couples like to use a blindfold to heighten their other senses. Without sight, they need to rely on sound, touch, and smell to locate their partner, what they are doing, and where they are going. It can make teasing even more fun when you have your hands tied above your head and your sense of sight taken away from you.

You can add to the sensory deprivation with noise-canceling headphones. It truly makes you rely on your sense of touch. Your world is dark and quiet, or dark and filled with music decided on by your partner, and your only connection is their hand on your hip as they thrust into you. Enjoy the feeling of being together rather than worrying about what you look like or what you sound like. You can't see or heard yourself anyway. Sensory deprivation is a great way to help yourself get lost in the moment, especially if you tend to get too in your own head and not focus on the pleasure. Use this as a chance to turn off your brain, don't worry too much about your common hang-ups, and just enjoy the fun.

Discipline Play

Discipline plays into the control based role-play. When one of you takes on the role of the dominant and the other the submissive, talk about what that means and what you want to do with it in the bedroom. Discipline play relies on setting up a set of rules for your submissive to follow, ways to enforce those rules, test the submissive's ability to follow the rules, and punishments when they don't follow them.

A common way of testing your submissive is orgasm control. The submissive is only allowed to orgasm when the dominant gives permission. This tactic is excellent for playing with edging. The more you get the submissive close to orgasm, the harder it will be to stave it off. If you add ways to heighten the sensations such as bondage or sensory deprivation, blindfolds, noise-canceling headphones, so that all they can focus on is how you are making them feel, it will be even more fun to tease them and get them to that point where they can't help but orgasm. If you haven't permitted them to do so, then you get to punish them.

Orgasm control is incredibly fun if you're playing around with it during penetrative sex. It takes quite a bit of focus to control your partner's orgasm and your own while you are teaching them self control. Vary the speed of your thrusts, how deeply you move. Use your partner's erogenous zones to your advantage to drive them wild and then back off. Remove all touch. Then start up again, faster than before, if you can manage it. See how many times you can get your partner close to the brink of orgasm before they finally disobey. Or reward them if they're obedient.

Punishment can take many forms, the most common being spanking. Pain and pleasure centers are linked closely in the brain. If we are in the right mindset, pain can feel very good and even heighten our pleasure. Many people find themselves to be more aroused when they are involved in consensual pain. Nipple clamps are a great addition as a punishment. You could either tighten them on your partner or tug on the attached string. Floggers are good because you can add stimulation to larger areas at a time. You can use the flogger on their thighs, chest, arms, and butt.

When it comes to those kinds of punishments, it's essential to know how much you can handle. Some people like to have their butt spanked cherry red. Other people get too sensitive after the first few spanks. Try it out before you're in the intense control role-play headspace and communicate using your colors if that's something you've decided to use beforehand. Communicate throughout, and have fun.

Punishments don't necessarily have to be painful. If you ordered your partner not to orgasm without permission, maybe keep giving them orgasms until they can't take it anymore, and they've reached hypersensitivity. Play with what makes you both feel good and do it just a few too many times as punishment. Be creative. Anything can be a punishment. It's up to you.

Games to Involve Your Whole Living Space
There are games you can play that incorporate your entire living space. House Party is a great example. The rules are simple. Neither of you gets to orgasm until you've had sex in every room of your apartment or house. Start where the mood takes you.

Maybe you're both inclined to have some fun immediately after dinner, and you want to start in the kitchen. Make sure everyone's comfortable and get going. But remember, no one orgasms.

Then move onto the living room. Let yourself cool down while you two watch a movie together and relax. Curl up in each other's arms and hold each other close, maybe tease each other while you're watching until you can't stand it anymore, and you go at it again. It'll be fun seeing how long you both can hold out if you can both hold out, and what to do with the first person who breaks the rules. The game is that much more fun if there is s a winner and a loser. Have the loser do something for the winner or have the winner get to punish the loser somehow.

From there, it's up to you. You can keep playing as before, keep having sex in different rooms of the house to see who can hold off on orgasm the longest and keep going until you've hit every room in the house. Or start entirely over again. Try to see if you can make it to each room before you orgasm.

Much like 'find the 'insert food item of your choice' game, you can play a version of this during sex. Have one partner blindfolded while the other picks from a variety of foods. Dab a bit of the food, such as chocolate sauce, whipped cream, ice cream, anything you can think of, on your finger, and let them lick it off. Or have them lick it off of any part of your body. You could do this with any food; it doesn't have to be a spreadable one. Make a fruit plate and have them try the different kinds of fruit. Now they guess. If they get it right, they get rewarded with some oral or a few thrusts. If they get it wrong, they get punished.

That's up to you to decide what the punishment will be. Will they be spanked? Will you remove all kinds of physical contact? Do whatever you want to make your partner squirm, then play another round.

Games to Play in the Bedroom

Similar to the no-hands game from earlier, where you do everything you possibly can to tease your partner without the use of your hands, this time, you'll try to do all that you can without using your hands while you're already naked. If the two of you decide that you want to have sex, how will you make that work without using your hands? You can use them to balance yourself, but you can't touch your partner.

Enjoy some oral without getting to run your fingers through your partner's hair. Hover your hands over your partner's breasts without actually touching them. Just let her feel the heat of your hand over her skin without any physical contact. This game is designed to help you two get creative with how you touch each other. What would usually seem like regular sex is now something completely different just by changing that one thing.

Try Not So Fast. This game can be played before, during, or after sex to make the aftercare a little more sensual. One of you will lie on the bed, ideally naked, and the other will stand in the doorway. The one lying on the bed will ask the other questions about them. What's their favorite ice cream flavor? Or What's the highest number of orgasms they've ever had at once? For every correct answer, the partner in the doorway gets to take a step forward. For every wrong answer, they take one step back. The better you two know each other, the less likely one of you will move so far back that you're in the kitchen. But it can be fun to make the questions hard so that they're not always walking forward toward you.

As they get closer, give them a little incentive to make it right to the bed. Start to tease yourself or show off how excited you are for them to win. When they do, you will surely make it worth their while.

Play this game in rounds. Maybe when the first partner makes it to the bed, that's not the end of the game. Keep track of how many questions it takes before each partner makes it to the bed. Whoever has to answer the least is the winner and can enjoy their spoils.

Use the timer from Red Light Green Light during sex. Set the timer and go at it until the timer goes off. Then you stop dead in your tracks; you don't move until you gather your bearings and set the timer again. Keep going, maybe switch positions each time you change position, and see who breaks and orgasms first. Or you can even make it a race. Instead of the first person to orgasm being the loser, make them the winner.

If you're switching positions each time the timer goes off, make it so that a different person is in control each time. That way, each time you run the timer, someone else is guiding the action and in control. Play around with speeds, depths, using toys, or not using toys. Have fun with it and do your best to make the other person orgasm as quickly as possible or as slowly as possible. It's up to you how you want to torment your partner.

Have a naked wrestling match. If you and your partner are of varying sizes, play with caution, and make sure you have safe words ready in case one of you should get too overpowered. But it can be fun to play with your whole body. Get naked or make this game part of getting each other unclothed. Wrestle each other on the bed or a nice carpeted surface, and once one of you has the other pinned, they get to do what they want until the other can break themselves free.

If you're playing this while getting naked, you'll have to be creative in how to keep your partner pinned and get their clothes off. All of the wriggling and squirming is a great way to get your partner aroused so that you can distract them use that to your advantage, and take over. Once you're both naked, then you can start with the real teasing and sex. See how long it takes for you to get your partner to give in and stop resisting your control.

Pull from your games from foreplay and see how you can make them work in the bedroom while you're going at it. You can mix up and combine the games however you see fit. Take Fatebowl. You each have your bowls of punishments or tasks for the other. Instead of rolling the dice to see what number will come up and see who loses, use sex as your determining factor. Make the rule that while you're having sex, you can't touch each other with your hands. Once one of you breaks that rule, they have to pick their fate. If they're lucky, their fate will continue the fun in the bedroom. And if they're unlucky, they're punishment will be to clean out the dishwasher. You can decide if you make them do that right now, effectively teasing the both of you so that you have to wait until they're finished to continue your play. Or they can do it later, and the two of you can continue playing, racking up punishments as you go along.

Try, Pick a Card. Take an ordinary deck of cards and assign each suit a different sexual act. Diamonds could be oral, spades could be hand job/fingering, clubs could be grinding, and hearts could mean penetration. Take turns drawing cards from the shuffled deck and perform those acts for the number value of seconds. You could do Ace high or Ace low. Just be warned that you may be getting a one-second hand job if your partner draws the ace of spades. For the face cards go up one value after ten—Jack for eleven, queen for twelve, and king for thirteen.

Whoever draws the card gets to perform the act. When it comes to penetration, the person drawing the card gets to drive the action, be in charge, be in control, and be on top. Either go through until you've run out the entire deck, or until you just can't stand it anymore and you have to keep going. There are only so many 4-second hand jobs someone can take before they pounce on their partner like a panther.

Mutual masturbation is a perfectly respectable form of sex. You both are enjoying yourself and watching the other enjoy themselves. It's fun, it's pleasurable, and if you're able to orgasm more than once or you're a man with a brief refractory period, it's a fun way to get things started once the clothes are off.

Make up some rules for yourselves, like you can't touch each other until one of you orgasms, or you can't move on to more sex until you've both reached orgasm. Have fun teasing each other while you masturbate together. Talk dirty to each other. Tell your partner what you plan to do to them once you've finished this round, and you're ready to move onto the next. Plan out a punishment for the person who orgasms second. Tell your partner what you're going to make them endure when they lose. Take your time to tease yourself slowly as you watch your partner. Show them how much fun you're having, and how much fun they'll be able to have after the game.

There's no wrong way to participate in mutual masturbation. All you two have to do is lie next to each other, sit nearby, or even stand across from each other and masturbate. Use your partner as your own personal porn.

Be your ideal porn. The mirror on the ceiling over the bed stereotype may be a bit extreme, but playing in front of a mirror can be very sexy. You get to see yourself getting aroused, your partner gets to watch you get turned on by watching both of you. It's very sensual. It can be fun to do a bit of mutual masturbation in front of the mirror. That way, you get to watch each other and yourselves, or just have sex in front of the mirror.

Try doggy style or reverse cowgirl. Both positions are covered in the next chapter. You can both watch yourself in the mirror or switch up positions to get a turn to watch yourself. If you have a mirror that you can move, put it close to the edge of the bed to get the full view. If you don't, try switching up the location where you're having sex to view yourself in the mirror you do have easily. If the only mirror you have in your bedroom is over a vanity or your dresser, use that to your advantage and have a little fun on a surface that isn't your bed. Or if the only mirror you have that's big enough to see both of you is the one in the bathroom, enjoy a little bathroom sex.

However you choose to play, the important thing is that you have fun with it. Sex is fun and messy and playful. You are allowed to laugh at how ridiculous it seems sometimes. Have fun with your partner and relax. The more relaxed you are, the more likely you will have fun with whatever you two choose to do together. Be sexy and most of all, have fun.

CHAPTER 9: POSITIONS

The position you're in can make a world of difference in the kind of sex you can have. Some positions lend themselves to calm, sweet lovemaking. Other positions tend to lean on the side of harder, rougher sex. You need to determine what is going to work for you and your partner.

The Basics

First, let us go over the basic positions and different variations that you can try to make them feel fabulous.

Missionary. Missionary is the 'traditional' sex position. The man is on top, and the woman is on the bottom. The term comes from the Christian missionaries as they thought that this position was more civilized. In the countries they were trying to spread their 'word of god' to, the other positions were considered more animalistic. As this was the position the missionaries encouraged in their converts, it became known as the missionary position.

Adding new elements to this position can make it feel that much more intense. Try adding some light bondage by binding your hands above your head or binding your legs so they stayed spread out. This gives your partner more access to enjoy your erogenous zones, and it gives you that delightful feeling of giving up control if that's something you want.

Play with the position of your legs. Instead of merely having them on the bed or your feet planted, wrap them around your partner while they thrust. Use your feet to guide their hips and lift your own hips to meet each thrust. This will help them stay closer and give you more control over the depth of the thrusts.

If you're flexible, try moving your legs up by your partner's shoulders. This position can give your partner the angle you need to move deeper and more likely to hit your g-spot as they move. If you're not that flexible, but still want that feeling, add some pillows or a wedge-shaped sex pillow you purchased until your hips lift it and let your partner get that extra angle.

Doggy Style. Having your partner penetrate you from behind can feel immensely pleasurable. It is one of the positions that makes it easier for you both to reach your clit. Reaching between you while your face to face can feel awkward for both of you, but with you on all fours and your partner penetrating you from behind, it's easy for them to reach your clit, it's easy for you to get your clit. It'll make the pleasure that much better.

You can also modify this with "Flat Doggy," where you lie on your stomach with your legs closed, and your partner penetrates you from behind. This will be pleasurable for them because of the added tightness that comes with your legs locked together, and this angle is useful for having your partner hitting your g-spot with their trusts. They're already angled for their thrusts to go slightly upward right into that spongey spot and make you feel fantastic.

Another variant of this is 'face down, ass up,' where you are on your knees, and instead of being up on your arms, your back is flat, your head is down against the pillows. This gives your partner more room to play and lifts your hips more so you both have better access to your clit. For some couples, this is more comfortable than the traditional doggy style due to their height differences. Play around with them and find what works best for you.

Spooning. Spooning can lead to very sensual sex. You get to feel your partner's body all over you as they drive you wild. There are a few ways you can accomplish this. Have your man behind you while you both lie on your side. Open your legs either by pulling your knee to your chest, and if you're flexible, try holding your leg up, or turn slightly onto your front and bend your leg a bit to create space for your partner.

Spooning sex can be slow and sweet or hard and fast. It's up to you. Like doggy style, this position is great for clit stimulation. It's much easier for your partner to wrap their arm around you and tease your clit, and you can rub your clit.

Spooning is also great if you like having your hands bound in front of you. Since your partner is behind you, they wouldn't be in the way of you two getting close. Additionally, you don't need to rely on your hands for balance like you would in doggy style because you're on your side.

This position is also great for hand jobs and fingering. This way, either of you can be the one behind the other, guiding the action. Enjoy the feeling of having your partner's whole body pressed up against you while they use their fingers to drive you wild. If you're partial to morning sex or waking the other up with a sexy surprise, this position is a great way to start. Press yourself against your partner, make yourselves warm and comfortable, and slowly tease them until they wake up and realize what you're doing.

Positions Where the Woman is On Top

Cowgirl. When you think about the woman being on top, the first position most people think of cowgirl. At its core, this position involves the woman on top of the man, guiding the action with her hips. This is an excellent position for female pleasure because it opens up the clit more for further stimulation from both of you. And if you bend over your partner, your clit is more likely to press against his pubic bone as you move.

While it looks like the woman is doing all of the work, the man should be doing his part. His hips should move with hers to deepen the thrusts. He can run his hands along his partner's body as she takes her pleasure on top of him. Grip her breasts, pinch her nipples, or suck on them if they're close enough to you. This position is not one-sided. No position should feel one-sided. You both should be doing your part to make sure the other is sufficiently turned on and satisfied.

Reverse Cowgirl. This position is what it sounds like, cowgirl but with the woman reversing the way she is faced. Her back is to the chest of her partner. This position is fun for many couples because of the view the partner on the bottom gets of you moving along their penis. It also allows you complete access to your clit as there is nothing in the way of you rubbing it in time with your thrusts.

Face Sitting. This is an excellent position for oral sex. If you have a headboard that you can grab onto or feel confident in your core strength, it's worth giving a try. As the name suggests, this position involves the man on his back with the woman straddling his face while he performs oral sex on her.

This position can be pleasurable because of the power dynamic involved. The woman can be driving the action, but she's ultimately at the mercy of her partner beneath her. It allows for a delicious push and pull of who has the control in this position. Typically, it is the woman. From here, she can grip her partner's hair, hold them close to her vulva. She can rock her hips more freely than she can be lying down. That feeling of being on top is intoxicating. There's a reason this position is also known as 'queening.' The woman is the queen, and the man's face is her throne. Embrace that power and give this position a try.

Standing Positions

Against the wall. One of the easiest, and safest, ways to try having sex standing up is to use the wall to your advantage. Have one partner against the wall while the other is having their way with you. You may need to open your legs more or prop one leg up on your partner's hip to ensure that you have enough space for your partner to do what they want with you. This can be extremely helpful if you two are of varying heights, and your vulva doesn't immediately line up with his penis. But most importantly, you need to keep your balance. This position can be fun, but it can also be dangerous if you don't have something close by to steady yourself. Just make sure that you are far from any dresser corners or counter edges so you won't bang your head if you lose your balance for a second.

Using the wall as a brace can also be useful if you're partner can lift you entirely. This can be a rough position and requires a lot of physical strength to keep up for long periods. You need to be able to both hold onto your partner for support and brace your back so you don't slam into it with every thrust. If this position appeals to you but seems too daunting or you're not sure you have the physical strength just yet, there are alternatives listed below.

On a counter. This position is a little bit of both seated and standing sex. The woman will be on the counter with her partner between her legs. This position is an excellent alternative if you want the change of scenery you'd get from standing sex while also having the added benefit of sitting down. You've taken out the danger element of losing your balance and give yourself a whole new surface to play on.

If you're playing on the counter in the bathroom, you can combine this with having sex in view of the mirror. If your partner faces the mirror as they thrust into you, they get to watch the two of you like their own personal porn. If you're able to use the side of the counter, now the two of you can watch yourselves in the mirror. It's a much bigger turn-on than most people give it credit.

If you're playing on the kitchen counter, you have easy access to play a game involving food while you have your fun. Either blindfold your partner and make them guess the food you've smeared over your hand or just have fun decorating your partner's body with chocolate sauce or whipped cream and enjoy licking it off as you have sex. It's hard to go wrong with this. You get sex and dessert.

Sex Swing. If you like the idea of sex against the wall, holding your partner up, but you don't have the physical strength just yet, this is where a sex swing could come in handy. As mentioned in the previous chapter about toys, sex swings are most commonly apparatuses that hang over the door's back and use the closed door to hold the whole thing up. Once you've situated your partner in the swing with her legs up and she feels secure, you could do anything you want to her.

From this angle, it's effortless to get down on your knees and perform oral sex on her, or you can have regular intercourse on it as well. Most swings are adjustable, so you don't have to worry about the one you have being the right height for you. And you don't have to worry about positioning your legs in the right place so that you fit together nicely. With a swing, you can just extend or shorten the straps that connect to the door anchors for your height and have fun with it.

These swings are suitable for standing sex, but they don't swing all that well. If you want a swing that operates more like a playground swing, you'll need to get a freestanding apparatus or something that can connect to the beam in your ceiling so that you have the full range of motion.

Mixed Positions

These positions involve one of you to be seated or lying down while the other is standing. One of the best positions like this for pleasure has the woman lying down with the man standing between her legs. You can either do this on your back or your stomach; it depends on the kind of sex you want to have.

Doing this position with the woman on her back leads to more sensual sex. It's very close to missionary, but you have more space between you. You can both get to your clit more quickly this way. This position can also lead to slightly rougher sex. When your partner is standing, it gives him more leverage to move his hips, thus allowing him to set any rhythm he wants, be that slow and sweet, or hard and fast. It's entirely up to the two of you.

If you're having sex in this position on your stomach, it can lead to rougher sex. It exposes your butt, so if you decided that spanking was something you wanted to try, this is a great way to incorporate it into your sex. You have more access to your clit this way, but if you position it just right, you can grind your clit against the bed itself with each thrust.

This position is good to use with some light bondage. If you're on your back, you can bind your hands above your head or in front of you. With them bound in front of you, it gives your partner a little bit of a handle to hold onto as they guide their thrusts. If you're on your front, you can once again bind them above your head or behind you, adding an extra feeling of helplessness and lack of control if that's something you decided you want.

It's simple enough to change up how you have sex. Take your go-to position and turn it 90 degrees or 180 degrees. Take missionary on its side, and now you have cuddling sex. Go a full 180 degrees, and now you have cowgirl. Even changing the angle the person on top holds themselves can make a big difference. See how you feel when you're close to your partner versus straightening your back and guiding the motion with your hips. The smallest changes can make a big difference when it comes to your pleasure.

Don't be afraid to try things that you might have otherwise been scared to do. If you want to try sex standing up, but you're fearful of the physical demands, find a modification. Use the counter as a seat, or try having sex while kneeling. Use a pillow to pad the floor and have fun. Buy a sex swing, so you get that full feeling of standing up without having to worry about holding your partner up. However you choose to adapt the position, if you're both into it, it'll always be fun.

No matter how you choose to have sex, enjoy the time with your partner. If you are face to face, enjoy the eye contact you can make with your partner or enjoy the eye contact you make through the mirror. Feel your partner's body against yours and how that added pressure makes you feel. Is it more comforting to feeling them against your back, or do you prefer to feel them pressed all against your front so you feel their body weight on you? Try out new positions and see what feels right to you. Don't be afraid to experiment. The worst that could happen is you stop and try a new position. Talk it out, tell each other when something is uncomfortable, or pinching you or your back is bothering you, and you need to switch. That's why safewords are there. Don't be afraid to use them, especially when you're trying out a new position.

Most importantly, have fun. Sex can be fun and games, it can be immensely pleasurable, and it can also go wrong. There's no harm in laughing off a bad experience and trying something new. It'll only bring you two closer together.

CHAPTER 10: AFTERCARE

Aftercare is crucial when it comes to connecting with your partner after sex. As the name would suggest, it is the care you give your partner after sex. It's the time for you two to calm down together, go over what you just did and how it made you feel, and what you want to do again.

Aftercare can be as simple as cuddling up together in the blankets and enjoying each other's company in the quiet after all of the fun. It can involve getting each other comfort items they may need or tending to their needs if it seems incredibly hard for them to come out of a scene. Ask them what they need, and do it. If they say they want you to hold them, hold them. If they say they want to take a shower, make sure they're okay to stand and help them into the shower.

If you two feel confident that your shower allows it and it won't further your arousal, take a shower together and get yourself clean. Sex is fun, but it's also exercise. You both are likely hot and sweaty, and it could feel nice to get that all washed off before you go to bed.

Aftercare is vital to discuss what you two just did and what you want to do again. If you were introducing a new toy, talk about how it made you feel. Did you like the placement or the strength of the vibrator? Did you try edging with it? How did you like it?

When you are of sound mind and less exhausted, go over your Want, Will, and Won't lists and look over the items you tried. Is anything moving to a different list? If you tried something on your Will list, like spanking, you found out you like, move it to your Want list. If you tried something on your Want list, like nipple clamps, and they did nothing for you and you have no desire to use them again, add them to your Won't list. Do this together so that you're both on the same page, and no one is bringing something up that was moved to one or the other's Won't list.

Massages

Massages aren't just fun as foreplay. They are essential to utilize during aftercare. Sex is exercise. You should treat it as such. After a good workout, what feels better than a good stretch and maybe a massage? Work out the sore muscles on your partner. If they were tied up, pay special attention to their shoulders. They're likely sore, stiff, and uncomfortable. Rub them in small, firm circles and watch your partner relax after your playtime.

Ask your partner where they are stiff. There's going to be at least one place where something got pulled, or they are feeling stiffer than when you started, even if you started with a massage. Give them what they need and help them relax. Tell your partner what's hurting you and if they're up for it, ask for a massage as well. You both had fun. You both deserve a little tender, loving care.

Cuddling

There is no better affective aftercare than cuddling, especially after a hot and heavy scene. Some people don't like contact after an intense scene, so talk that through with your partner. But if you both are okay with it. Cuddle close under a warm blanket, maybe some fresh sheets if you're still in bed, and get comfortable. This is the perfect time to get close to each other and talk about what you did if you can both make words. For some people, it takes a little while before they can get out of the headspace they were in during sex and become a regular person again. Take your time and relax with your partner while you come down from the high of all of the hormones and adrenaline previously coursing through your body.

Cuddling increases the body's level of Oxytocin. It can sometimes act as a pain reliever, which can be useful for your sore muscles, and releases through a positive feedback system in the brain. It releases during arousal, sex, and aftercare while cuddling with your partner. Sometimes it is known as the 'love hormone,' often being released in times of bonding. This hormone can help make your connection to your partner seem that much stronger.

Take as much time as you need just to cuddle and hold your partner. Enjoy that feeling of closeness and warmth with them. Take in their scent. It might seem strange, but many people find inhaling their partner's scent or musk to be very calming for them, especially after sex.

When you're ready to talk, do so with an open mind and open ears. Listen to your partner. Something might be bothering them now that you're done. There may be something you were eager to try again that they don't want to ever think about doing. Talk it through. You don't have to go through the last few hours with a fine-toothed comb. But talk about the big things you added. The new games you got from this book that you wanted to try. Talk it out.

Be patient. Not every chance to try new things is going to be a slam dunk. You're not going to like every single new thing you try. And that's okay. It's more important to weed out what you don't like. You have to crack a few eggs if you're going to make an omelet. There are bound to be flops that you thought would be amazing that after trying them, you decide you never want to try them again. As long as you're honest with your partner, there's no harm in having tested. You took the air of mystery out of the act.

If there are items you're unsure about, a toy you tried for the first time, a different position, or a new kind of role-play game, those are even more important to talk through. There's some gray area, some wiggle room, to see where you can make it better. It's not a hard and fast no, never again, but it's also not a quick and excited absolutely. You have to figure out what you can change with your partner so that you can both enjoy it more.

If you tried control-based role-play with one set of roles, but they didn't really fit, try it again. This time you're the dominant, and your partner is the submissive. See how differently the same game can feel just by changing one thing. If the issue was the vibrator you used, maybe from your angle, it was uncomfortable to hold. Perhaps next time, your partner can try holding it. It would give the vibrator a new angle, and it would free up your hand to do something else.

Talk about your safe word system. Did you like it? Did you feel that you were in a position where you could freely say the word or color you needed to if the time came? Discuss if you need to change the safe word to something else. Maybe one of you said it, and it wasn't clear enough. It's always best to choose a word that would never come up in a sex game scenario. You never want your safe word to be something that could easily be mistaken for an exclamation of enjoyment. Keeping the system clear with colors is the easiest way to avoid this confusion. If you tried a safe word and didn't like how it felt, try the color system next time.

Did a situation come up where you felt like you needed to use your safe word? Talk that through. The rope holding you to the bed was too tight, and you felt like you were losing circulation in your hands. The things your partner was saying while in character were starting to feel too real and personal, and you wanted them to take a step back with it. Something involving the sex was painful, and you didn't know what. These are all valid reasons to say your safe word. There is no invalid reason to use your safe word. It's there to keep you safe. If anything at all strikes you as painful, hurtful, or not fun, sat it as clearly as you can so that your partner hears you and can stop what they're doing.

When you talk with your partner, and there is that mutual trust there, you feel much freer to discuss your wants and desires. As you explore new areas of your sexuality, it'll be that much easier to find new things you want to try, new things you are willing to try, and yes, some things you won't try or won't do again. It's part of the exploration. You find the good in with the bad. As long as the bad is done safely, you never have to worry about getting hurt.

Take a Bath Together

It may seem a little counterintuitive to get close and naked with each other after you were just close and naked together, but it can be fun for some couples. Sex is hot and sweaty, and there are a lot of bodily fluids everywhere. Getting clean after sex is just as important as it can be fun and comforting.

If you have a big enough bathtub to hold the two of you, draw a warm bath, and get comfortable. Maybe have one of you lie between the other's legs so you're chest to back. If you have bubbles, you can incorporate those, or add in some scented bath salts. Do whatever you need to relax. This is aftercare. The goal is relaxation. Take the time to enjoy feeling your partner pressed against you as the warm water surrounds you and relaxes your muscles.

You still need to get clean, so let your partner lather up some body wash in their hands or on a loofa and enjoy the feeling of their hands against your skin. If you want to turn this into more play, there's no harm in that. You're in a hot, sensual position. It makes sense that you'd want to further the intimacy. If you decide to have some fun in the bathtub or shower, remember that water washes away everything, including natural vaginal lubricants. Use a silicone-based lubricant to make up for this. Water-based lube will wash out in the water, just like your natural lubricants.

If you don't have a bathtub or your tub isn't big enough to hold the both of you, try taking a shower together. Not only does it have all of the added benefits of a bath, the warm water, being close to your partner, and the potential for more play. But it also has the bonus of not making you feel too cramped. Even the most spacious bathtubs can feel a bit small when there are two adults in it.

When it comes to enjoying the shower together, if you decide to get frisky in there, use silicone-based lubricant and make sure your feet stay on the floor to make sure everyone is safe. Intimacy in the shower can be fun, but the slick surfaces can make it dangerous. Proceed with caution.

If you're just using the shower as a cool down, focus on getting clean. Scrub each other down, wash each other's hair, and enjoy the closeness with your partner while you get clean. Enjoy your nighttime routine together. It'll extend the intimacy through your bedtime routine until you can get back into bed together and relax for the night.

Cooling Down After Sex

Aftercare is all about cooling down and bringing your body back into a state of relaxation. Cuddling and getting clean is essential, but so can just being with the other person. It doesn't mean you have to interact or wholly against the other. But if you're in the same bed together, relaxing, maybe one of you is watching a video on their phone, and the other is reading a book, or you're just watching something together, you're spending that time close to them after you've had a fun night and are ready to wind down to get some sleep.

Read together. Reading together can mean you are beside each other, reading separate books, or it can mean that one of you is reading aloud while the other listens. This gives you something you can do together with little movement. Just lie together and enjoy the quiet or the sound of your voice as you narrate the story. Hopefully, this is soothing for both of you. You can trade off who is reading aloud if that's the route you want to go. You can each take over a character voice. Or just one of you can read aloud while the other listens. Whichever works for your partnership. One of you may be more inclined to listen, while the other prefers to do the reading. We all relax differently.

Like watching a movie or tv show together before sex, watching something together after sex can be an excellent way to wind down for the night and relax in your partner's arms. Don't pick anything that will get you too excited. Just watch something light that you both enjoy and relax your mind after all of that work you put in during sex.

Sex is not only exercise; it can also be very mentally draining. Finding a way to relax your mind afterward is just as important as relaxing the muscles in your body. Rewatch an old favorite on the streaming service of your choice, or something saved on your DVR, and enjoy the warmth of your partner as you relax for the night.

Plan for Next Time

Planning can be done during your cuddles and getting ready for bed, or it can be the next morning, afternoon, or even the week after. Talk about what you liked about the new things you tried, or old standards you used, and how they made you feel. Talk about your likes and dislikes. If there's a game that you tried for the first time that you really liked. If you both enjoyed it and want to try it again, see if there's anything on your list that invokes a similar feeling or think might be pleasurable in a similar way.

Say you tried playing Red Light Green Light during your foreplay. You liked using the timer; you thought it was fun to have that time constraint on you as you played. If that's something you both enjoyed, maybe next time you can play Pick a Card and use that next time as your foreplay and play Red Light Green Light during your penetrative sex.

If you found a toy that you liked, figure out what it was about it that you enjoyed. Was it the vibration or the size? Was it the ease of use during sex? Discuss buying more toys like it. It's always a good idea to have various toys so that you are never bored with your bedroom options. When it doubt, grab a toy out of the box.

Look over your Want, Will, and Won't lists and discuss what you want to move around. If you tried something on your Will list, like spanking, is that something you want to move to your Want list? Did the way you two tried it, making sure it was with an open hand or that your partner only spanked you during intercourse, make you more inclined to try it in the future? Did you hate it? Maybe it did nothing for you, and you have no desire to be spanked ever again. Or perhaps you're still indifferent to it. You liked it enough, your partner liked it, but your opinion on being spanked didn't change at all. Move it to the appropriate list or leave it where it is.

If something happened during your playtime that prompted one of you to use your safe word, talk it through. Figure out if that aspect of your play, maybe it was bondage with rope, should be removed from your arsenal going forward. You really didn't like the rope's feeling and how it made you feel when you were tied down. There was no way to adjust it so that you were comfortable. You don't see a way to make bondage with rope something you can add back into the bedroom anytime soon. Talk to your partner not only about how it felt physically, but how it felt mentally. If the issue was primary physical, you could always try with another material or a different position. But if it was mental, there may not be a way to modify the action so you are both comfortable. Talk it through, see if there is a middle ground, should you need to find one, and see where you land. You may not be able to find a middle ground, and that is okay. Keep moving down your Want, Will, and Won't lists and discover other items you can try next time.

Aftercare isn't just the moment after you're finished with sex. Just like how foreplay can extend throughout your entire day, so can aftercare. All it means is that you are both taking care of each other's needs after sex. It helps you feel closer and extend your intimacy after sex. You can do this no matter where you are. Attending to each other's mental and physical needs does not end at the bedroom door. It should extend to your entire relationship. It consists of the three C's: comfort, communication, and care. Comfort each other and work out your sore and achy muscles. Communicate about your desires and boundaries after the fact. And care for each other in any way you possibly need. Spicing up your bedroom time can be taxing on the mind. Take the time to care for yourself and your partner. Make sure you always feel the love.

CONCLUSION

Hopefully, this book has been helpful for you, and you walk away from it with some new ideas on how to add some extra fun to your bedroom time. If you've done your homework, you should have Want, Will, and Won't lists that are teeming with ideas to get you started talking with your partner. Maybe you even have a few new kinks you didn't know you had before you started.

The number one thing to take away from this book is: communication is critical. You cannot have good sex without communication. Vanilla or kinky, missionary or doggy style, you need to feel comfortable talking to your partner about your wants and desires, and when things go wrong, and you want to change things up.

Maybe you have some new techniques to help you reach orgasm in the bedroom, and now you're not so ashamed to admit that it doesn't always happen with your partner. Now you know how good it can feel when you both can get there, and you both enjoy the look on the other's face when they do. Orgasms are fun, simple, and effective ways of showing your partner you care about their sexual wellbeing, but it's not the only way.

Now you know the importance of aftercare and what it can do for your relationship. Spending more time attending to each other's needs after sex will help bring the two of you closer together in ways you didn't know possible. Hold each other close, talk things out, and make a plan for next time.

With these tools, you can make your sex life that much more satisfying and loving. Be open, be kind, be loving. And most importantly. Don't forget to have as much fun as you possibly can.